THE VITAMINS EXPLAINED SIMPLY

A guide to what vitamins are, what they do and their importance in our diet.

D0784784

THE VITAMINS EXPLAINED SIMPLY

Prepared and produced by the Editorial Committee of Science of Life Books

Revised and Extended by
Leonard Mervyn B.Sc., PhD., F.R.S.C.

SCIENCE OF LIFE BOOKS
4-12 Tattersalls Lane, Melbourne, Victoria 3000

Seventh Edition, revised, enlarged
and reset, February 1984
Second Impression June 1984

© SCIENCE OF LIFE BOOKS 1984

*Registered at the G.P.O. Sydney
for transmission through the
post as a book*

British Library Cataloguing in Publication Data

Mervyn, Leonard
    The vitamins explained simply.
    1. Vitamins in human nutrition
    I. Title
    613.2'8   TX553.V5

    ISBN 0-909911-07-X

National Library of Australia card number
and ISBN 0 909911 07 X

Printed in Great Britain by
Richard Clay (The Chaucer Press) Ltd,
Bungay, Suffolk

Contents

Foreword

Never before has there been a greater need for correct, clear and concise information about vitamins. Vitamins are food factors, essential micro nutrients which enter into many biochemical reactions within the body, enabling us to make better use of the food we eat. Without an adequate daily intake of vitamins the whole biochemistry of the body is upset. Each vitamin has a specific area of influence and must be supplied in adequate amounts to meet individual needs.

It is very true that 'All men are not born equal', particularly where nutrition is concerned and today we know that not only does our occupation and life style influence our nutritional requirements but also our genetic or hereditary background. A few years ago conditions known as 'Vitamin Dependency Syndromes' were recognized, in which it was found that through genetic influences some individuals had a higher than normal requirement for one or more of the vitamins. If these people did not receive considerably more of the particular vitamin concerned than the amount required by the average person, they developed deficiency symptoms although their dietary intake was adequate according to accepted standards.

Like other nutrients in our diet vitamins are absorbed from the small intestine some 2½ to 6 hours after eating. The major site of absorption is in the first half of the small intestine where 90 per cent of all absorption takes place. The critical period for absorption is some 2½ to 4½ hours after eating. Vitamin B_{12} is an exception, absorption taking place in the lower end of the small intestine some six hours after eating. To ensure maximum absorption Vitamin tablets or capsules should break down and disintegrate in the stomach so that the contents are ready for absorption when the food reaches the small intestine. 'Slow release' or 'delayed release' vitamins with a release time longer than four hours are of doubtful value.

Some vitamins such as the fat soluble vitamins can be stored in the body, others such as vitamin C are not. Since vitamins help us to get the most out of our food it is only reasonable to take our vitamins with our food and where supplements in the form of tablets or capsules are being used, to determine the daily dosage required, divide this figure by three and then take ⅓ of the daily dosage with each meal. It can be false economy to take the whole daily dosage at one time, particularly where vitamins are being used for therapeutic purposes. For example it may be desirable to take 10,000mg vitamin C per day for a few days to help overcome an attack of flu or to fight off a cold. The maximum amount of vitamin C which can be absorbed from the small intestine at any one time is 3,000mg so that if 10,000mg were to be taken at one time, at least 7,000mg will not be absorbed through normal biochemic pathways. What happens to it? We are not certain but it is very likely eliminated rapidly through the kidneys and the bowels. In this case 3,000mg taken three times daily at regular intervals would be far preferable to 10,000mg taken in one large dose.

It is not uncommon to find some people who think that they can substitute vitamin tablets for food. This misconception has been brought about by incorrect information from various sources, vitamin supplements cannot be used to replace food and they are not intended to do so, they are invaluable however in making good deficiencies due to an inadequate diet or to other causes.

The diet of many people today leaves much to be desired and most people appear to be motivated by palate tempting dishes, convenience foods and take away foods of dubious nutritional value rather than by food of high nutritive value.

Perhaps the biggest nutritional enemies we face are alcohol and white sugar. An excessive amount of each is consumed in our 'Western diet'. Both of these so called foods contain no vitamins, moreover they increase the need for B group vitamins. However they both have the effect of satisfying the appetite and reducing the intake of nutritious vitamin rich foods. This means that on one hand they increase the need for vitamins and on the other hand they effectively reduce vitamin intake from food. It is little wonder that under the influence of our 'Western' lifestyle vitamin deficiencies are much more widespread than would appear.

A few years ago in Western Australia where there is an abundance of 'good food' available 3721 people were hospitalized in one year due to vitamin or other nutritional deficiencies. There are no statistics available however for those suffering from marginal deficiencies not requiring hospital treatment.

In another study it was shown that 10.7 per cent of a sample of 210 women were below the lower limit of the reference range for vitamin B_6.

In South Australia another study showed that 25 per cent of pregnant women taking part were deficient in folic acid.

Another survey conducted in a Sydney suburb showed that one third of the children in the area failed to reach the recommended daily intake for at least one nutrient.

There are many more similar studies available. These few however give an indication of the extent of marginal deficiencies in our community. Marginal vitamin deficiencies are much more widespread in our society than is generally recognised. There is a great need for nutritional education, particularly concerning the value of vitamins and the important role they play in nutrition.

It is essential to remember that vitamins are constituents of whole natural foods and that when deficiencies have developed, these have usually occurred following a sub-optimal intake over a period of months or sometimes years. Such deficiencies can seldom be corrected overnight and it is frequently necessary to take vitamins for from three to six months or even longer before there is much noticeable improvement. Vitamins should always be used along with a corrective diet as part of the overall nutritional programme. In some cases improvement may begin after a few days, however this is the exception rather than the rule and many people have become disheartened because they did not receive the immediate miraculous results they expected. These people tend to regard vitamins in the same manner in which they consider drugs. Vitamins are not 'remedies' they are absolute nutritional necessities without which the body cannot function normally. Adequate amounts must be obtained either from food or from supplementary sources if deficiencies are to be avoided.

This book is designed to give the reader a better appreciation of each individual vitamin, what the deficiency symptoms of each individual vitamin are and the way in which we can intelligently use vitamins both in foods and as food supplements to assist in the maintenance and restoration of health.

WILLIAM KING D.O., D.C.
New South Wales

1

What Vitamins Are

During the nineteenth century, various research workers recognized, from experience gained with scurvy, rickets, and beri-beri, that there were certain unknown factors in food, capable of preventing these diseases.

Experiments were conducted to ascertain what the mysterious food factors were. In these experiments, all the then known constituents of food, namely, re-purified fat, protein, carbohydrates, mineral salts and water were fed to laboratory animals under test conditions.

Prof. J.C. Drummond, in *The Englishman's Food*, says:

There was a good deal of interest about that time in the function in the body of the various mineral salts derived from food. Prof. Bunge of the University of Basle, Switzerland, was particularly interested in the subject and in 1881 he encouraged a young Russian assistant, N. Lunin, to attempt to rear young mice on food mixtures that had been so purified that they contained very small residual traces of mineral salts. Not surprisingly, he found that they survived a very short time.

. . . Finally he added the whole of the mineral ash of milk, thinking that by doing so he would be supplying all the necessary minerals. To his surprise the results were no better . . . .

Side by side with these cases of mice were others containing animals fed on milk itself. The animals flourished.

Bunge asked the question, 'Does milk contain, in addition to protein, fat and carbohydrates, other organic substances which are indispensable to the maintenance of life? It would be worth while to continue the experiment'. Unfortunately, Bunge did not do so . . . . He was on the very threshold of the discovery of vitamins, for it was by almost identical experiments that 25 years later, Pekelharing, Stepp, and Hopkins independently got evidence of the existence of a new class of dietary essentials.

There seems little doubt that the discoveries by Louis Pasteur in the realm of microbiology, made public about that time, unwittingly steered many scientists away from the real cause of scurvy, rickets and beri-beri, namely, vitamin deficiencies, so that instead of searching for vitamins they were looking for microbes.

Vitamin Research Continues

The word 'vitamin' was coined by the Polish chemist Casimir Funk in 1911. He extracted from rice polishings a crystalline substance capable of curing beri-beri and named it 'vita-amine', meaning essential to life and health and containing basic or 'amine' nitrogen. Subsequently, the final 'e' was omitted and the word became 'vitamin'.

Up to the present, over twenty different vitamins have been isolated and more are being investigated.

Research has proved that food contains minute quantities of substances required for normal growth and the maintenance of health. These substances are now known to be vitamins, which may be defined as essential food accessories.

The Quantities We Need

Compared to the amounts of the main constituents of food such as protein, carbohydrate, fats and fibre, the quantities of vitamins present are minute and it is pertinent to consider why these micro nutrients exert such a profound effect upon the health of the body. Even within the vitamins themselves there are vast variations in the quantities required to maintain health. The daily requirements of vitamin C, for example, are at least 30 mg but those of vitamin B_{12} are much lower at only 3 mcg. We need ten thousand times more vitamin C than vitamin B_{12} on a weight basis yet the manifestation of deficiency of either vitamin is equally serious and in both cases will ultimately result in death. Our daily requirements for the vitamins reflect the quantities present in a good, mixed, balanced and varied diet so we must assume that over the millions of years that human beings have evolved, the body's processes have adapted to the amounts of these micro nutrients fed to it daily. Hence it would be impossible for the diet to supply, for example, even as little as 1 milligram (1000 microgrammes) of vitamin B_{12} without eating at least 1 kilogram (2.2 pounds) of ox liver daily. On the other hand, according to Dr

Linus Pauling in his book *Vitamin C and the Common Cold* (1970) it would not be impossible for an adult person to receive 2.3 grammes of vitamin C daily from a chosen acceptable diet, a quantity some eighty times greater than the minimum daily recommended allowance in the UK. Yet medical research has indicated that some people are not receiving even the 30 mg of vitamin C needed daily and others are deprived of the minute amount of 3 cg vitamin B_{12} necessary.

Why Vitamins are Essential

The reasons why vitamins are essential lie in the basis of life itself. The process of life depends upon thousands of chemical reactions that are going on in every living creature, plant or animal or micro-organism, every second of every day. These chemical transformations would be too slow to sustain life if it were not for accelerators or living catalysts known as enzymes.

Enzymes are required to digest the food we eat to enable it to be absorbed and utilized by the body. Enzymes are necessary to convert that digested food into energy that is utilized in so many ways. We need energy for muscle contraction; for building up body tissues in the repair of the body from the wear and tear that is produced by everyday living; for warding off disease; for proper functioning of the essential organs and in maintaining a healthy brain and nervous system. Enzymes are also essential in the many transformations and interconversions amongst body substances that are a feature of normal metabolism.

Every body function therefore depends upon an

efficient enzyme system. Enzymes are therefore the basis of life itself. However, in order to function effectively, enzymes in turn require other substances to be present to make them go. These substances are known as enzyme cofactors or coenzymes and in many cases they are vitamins. Hence without the presence of a coenzyme, which is usually a vitamin, the enzyme does not function. When the enzyme ceases working, the appropriate body function it is stimulating slows down or stops and the end result is illness and eventually death.

It is therefore not difficult to see how vitamins are essential to maintain life. The body can make the enzymes we require from the food we eat. It cannot make the vitamins so these can only be supplied ready-made in the diet.

Factors Influencing the Utilization of Vitamins

Availability: Not all of the vitamins in a food may be available for absorption. One example is that much of the nicotinic acid (vitamin B_3) in cereals is bound as an insoluble complex. It cannot become available for absorption in the intestine unless the cereal is previously treated with alkali. Fat-soluble vitamins may fail to be absorbed if the digestion of fat is impaired. When mineral oils such as liquid paraffin are used consistently as laxatives, they are capable of dissolving the fat-soluble vitamins from the food and hence make them unavailable for absorption.

Provitamins: These are substances that occur in foods which are not themselves vitamins but are capable of being converted to vitamins by the body itself. Thus the carotenes are provitamins (precursors) of vitamin A; nicotinic acid can be produced from the amino acid tryptophane and vitamin D is synthesized in the skin by the action of sunlight on certain skin fats produced from cholesterol.

Production within the intestine: The normal 'friendly' bacteria that inhabit the lower part of the intestine are capable of synthesizing significant amounts of certain vitamins. These include vitamin K, nicotinic acid, riboflavin, vitamin B_{12}, folic acid and biotin. Unfortunately in most people some of these vitamins are produced too far down the gut to be absorbed, but it is likely that a significant part of our daily needs of vitamin K and biotin is supplied in this manner. When there is a too large population of bacteria present in the gut as in diarrhoea, they are more likely to reduce the amounts of vitamins available from the food. This is because the bacteria extract vitamins from the ingested food and retain them until they are excreted in the faeces.

Interaction of nutrients: An increased intake of starchy foods, sugars or alcohol requires an increased amount of vitamin B_1 to cope with them. Similarly if the diet is rich in polyunsaturated fatty acids such as vegetable oils and margarines, the requirement for vitamin E is also increased. Because of this interaction the nutritive value of a diet in respect of a specific vitamin may be less than that expected from an analysis of its contents, so a mild deficiency can develop.

What Vitamins There Are
The vitamins are divided into two groups, namely, the water-soluble vitamins which comprise the

vitamin B complex and vitamin C. The vitamin B complex is comprised of B_1, B_2, B_6, B_{12}, nicotinic acid (known also as B_3), pantothenic acid (known also as B_5), folic acid, biotin and arguably choline and inositol. The fat-soluble vitamins are A, D, E and K.

Fat-soluble vitamins require that some fatty foods be eaten to ensure their assimilation. Once assimilated, however, they can be stored within the body. The water-soluble vitamins by virtue of their solubility are not stored to any great extent in the body so they are readily excreted and must be replaced daily.

How a Vitamin is Defined

There are no absolutely clear-cut definitions of vitamins but the following criteria are a guide. Such criteria are important because often new nutrients are isolated and claimed to be vitamins when later studies indicate that this is not so.

To be a true vitamin a substance must satisfy these criteria:

1 It must be available only from the food and be unable to be produced within the body in sufficient amounts for health.
2 Its deficiency must induce specific clinical symptoms.
3 These symptoms must clear up on treating with the substance.

Hence although choline and inositol are loosely regarded as being B vitamins, they are not strictly so by virtue of their synthesis within the body cells.

However, modern research suggests that the body may not be able to manufacture sufficient of these substances for its uses under certain conditions, so a food supply then becomes important.

The Potencies of Vitamins

Strictly speaking we should be able to derive all our needs of vitamins from the food we eat, but unfortunately this hypothetical concept does not often work out in practice. Reasons are varied but they include: (i) losses during cooking of food; (ii) losses during storage of food; (iii) inability to absorb vitamins from the food. In addition, people vary in their individual requirements for vitamins and certain factors can increase our requirements, amongst which are: (i) stress; (ii) taking medicinal drugs, and (iii) habits like smoking and drinking. The effects of all of these factors on individual vitamins will be discussed in turn. However, because of these factors we can look at vitamin intake under three headings:

1   A biochemical intake — the minimum amount we require to ensure sufficient for normal body processes.
2   A 'topping-up' intake — a higher amount to satisfy increased requirements induced by the factors mentioned above.
3   A therapeutic intake — large amounts needed to treat a condition where the vitamin is acting like a medicinal drug rather than a food constituent.

A good, varied and balanced diet will ensure (1) and a carefully chosen diet may enable (2) to be satisfied, but (3) without doubt requires high-potency vitamins in tablet or capsule form since it is impossible to obtain such high quantities from the diet alone. It is for these reasons that vitamins are available in such a wide range of potencies and we shall discuss their merits under individual headings.

2

Vitamin A

In a series of experiments carried out between 1906 and 1912, British biochemist Garland Hopkins showed that young rats fed casin (pure milk protein), starch, sugar, lard and mineral salts failed to grow and eventually died. The addition to this diet of only 3 cc of milk daily enabled the rats to thrive. Thus was demonstrated the existence of an 'accessory food factor' in milk. In 1913, two groups of American researchers extracted this 'accessory food factor' from butter and from egg yolk and cod liver oil. Two years later, one of these groups — two researchers called McCollum and Davis — proposed the name 'fat-soluble A' to distinguish the factor from 'water-soluble B' that they had detected in whey, yeast and rice polishings. Eventually the name was reduced simply to Vitamin A.

Long before its isolation it had been known that there was a substance in liver that was beneficial in certain eye diseases. In 1904, Mori treated conjunctivitis in Japan by giving cod liver oil. It was noted too, during Hopkins' experiments, that young rats fed his special diet deficient in milk and butter developed conjunctivitis. It is not surprising therefore to find that one of the fundamental functions of vitamin A is in maintaining healthy sight and eyes.

Where Vitamin A Functions

Research has revealed that vitamin A has special functions relating both to the skin and that inner covering known as the epithelium. The latter lines the inside of the mouth, nose, sinuses, throat, bronchial tubes, air passages in the lungs, stomach, intestines, gall bladder, urinary bladder, kidney tubules, mastoids, inner ear, also the inner surface of the eyelids and conjunctiva.

Laboratory tests with animals have shown that when their diets are adequate in all respects except for vitamin A, they develop infections in some or other parts of the body already mentioned. Other test animals fed adequate vitamin A remained free from these infections.

Dr Wolbach of Harvard School of Medicine, has shown that when there is a deficiency of vitamin A, the cells forming the epithelium multiply at a faster rate than normal. When these cells die, they become hard and dry. Other cells growing beneath them, push them upwards and they too die, so that presently there are layers of dry, dead cells, as occurs with dandruff.

Work of Healthy Cells

Healthy cells of the epithelium secrete a moisture that keeps growth normal, but dead cells do not. The surface of the dry cells is therefore not washed clean with mucus, but is roughened and retains bacteria in an environment favourable to their rapid growth, that is, where there is food available for them in warm, sheltered surroundings. These bacteria exude enzymes (ferments) which are toxic to the body and the enzymes break down the body's cellular structure.

Healthy cells, on the other hand, produce anti-enzymes, which destroy the enzymes released by bacteria. One of these anti-enzymes, lysozyme, is contained in the mucus secretion found in the nose and also in tears, and has a strong antiseptic action.

After vitamin A had been added to the diet of laboratory animals previously deprived of this vitamin, healthy changes in the epithelium were observed within five days. In human beings, such changes take longer, depending upon the severity of the vitamin A deficiency.

In the early days of research into Vitamin A it became popularly known as the 'anti-infective vitamin', because lack of it lowered the resistance of animals and man to disease. It now appears likely that although the vitamin may contribute directly to warding off disease, its main function lies in maintaining a healthy skin and mucous membranes, so ensuring that the body's first barriers to attack by bacteria and viruses are intact.

Vitamin A and Internal Organs

In certain diseases, namely, those affecting the liver and kidneys, the intestines, also pneumonia, bronchitis, and other ailments of the respiratory system, the body's requirements of vitamin A are greatly increased and its reserves are rapidly exhausted. Here, however, infections and other diseases are actually creating deficiency of the vitamin. If sufficient of the nutrient is not supplied to overcome this induced deficiency, resistance is lowered further and a vicious circle results. Fortunately the liver is the great storehouse of vitamin A and as long as ample reserves are present the increased requirements needed are met from these.

Vitamin A Functions and the Eye

As far as the eye is concerned, vitamin A functions in maintaining healthy eye tissues as well as in the process of light itself.

We have seen that in deficiency of the vitamins, epithelial cells undergo changes whereby they become flattened and heaped upon one another. When this happens in the conjunctiva (the mucous membrane covering the eyeball) a condition called xerophthalmia develops. Xerophthalmia means literally dry eye. Whilst confined to the conjunctiva, this condition has no effect on the sight but it does tend to cause the eyeball to protrude giving rise to 'pop-eyes'. As the deficiency gets worse, this condition spreads to the transparent part of the eyeball, the cornea, and once this is affected blindness results. Young children between the ages of three and four years are the most susceptible to this aspect of vitamin A deficiency. Single lack of vitamin A remains the number one cause of blindness in the world today.

Vitamin A is essential for vision in dim light. It is well known that when entering a darkened room from a bright area, there is a short period when one is literally blind. In a few seconds, however, the eyesight becomes adapted to the dark conditions and objects become discernible. The time required to adapt to this night vision is lengthened when vitamin A is deficient and the condition is known as night blindness. Night blindness is a recognized symptom of vitamin A deficiency. There is a substance in the retina of the eye called rhodopsin (visual purple) upon which normal night vision depends. When light enters the eye some visual purple is used up and the products of such destruction bring about nerve impulses which inform the brain what the eye sees.

Replacements of visual purple, which is composed of vitamin A and protein, are normally conveyed by the bloodstream to the eye to make good the losses mentioned, but if the body's intake of vitamin A is deficient, there is a diminished supply of visual purple and this gives rise to dim vision in a poor light, or night blindness.

When sties form on the eye, or corneal ulcers occur, they are indications of a vitamin A deficiency. Severe burning and itching eyes often lack vitamin A.

Those who are over-sensitive to light or glare, may be in need of vitamin A and many people who find it necessary to wear sun glasses are probably deficient in this vitamin.

Other Manifestations of Vitamin A Deficiency

When the diet is low in vitamin A, the hair becomes dry and coarse and the scalp itchy. The hair lacks lustre and may begin to fall out; dandruff generally forms on the scalp and the nails become brittle, peel, or break easily.

The effect of a vitamin A shortage upon the skin is very noticeable. The pores become clogged with dead cells because the skin's oil glands are not functioning properly. The pores gradually develop blackheads, whiteheads, pimples and other skin blemishes. The skin on the back of the forearm, also the elbows, knees, buttocks and thighs develops small, horny spines. Unhealthy skin, due to this cause, is susceptible to boils, carbuncles and impetigo. Cysts may also form around such dead cells.

Practically all the body's supply of vitamin A is stored in the liver, the small remainder being held in the kidneys and lungs. Excess carotene is stored in the liver and fatty tissue below the skin.

Babies store relatively less vitamin A than adults and Dr Wolbach considers this is why they so frequently suffer from skin rashes and infections. He states that babies should be given fish liver oil from the first week of birth, instead of waiting until the sixth or eighth week.

Vitamin A's Many Uses

Adequate vitamin A is necessary for normal growth, for the formation and preservation of healthy bone structure, the integrity of the enamel of the teeth, good appetite and the normal production of red and white blood cells. It is needed also, as we have seen, for healthy skin and mucous membrane, and for good sight. A dry mouth may indicate a lack of vitamin A. This vitamin is also considered to delay the aging process and to promote long life.

It has been found that stored vitamin A becomes more effective if up to 100 mg of vitamin E is taken daily. This is because vitamin E functions as a protective agent for vitamin A, both in foods and within the digestive system and body tissues.

Daily Requirements

A baby should be given up to 1000 International Units of vitamin A daily from birth and a growing child up to 2000 units daily. An adult requires approximately 2500 units a day to ensure good health.

The dosage for elderly people can be up to double the adult dosage, because one's requirements of vitamin A increases with age.

The mother who breast-feeds her baby has greater requirements of 4000 IU daily during the first six months, according to UK recommendations.

In sickness, the dosage may also call for more than the daily intake, and some eye ailments need an increased dosage until the trouble is overcome. However, only under medical supervision should the daily supplement of vitamin A exceed 7500 IU.

UK government legislation now insists that vitamin A should be expressed in foods and dietary supplements as microgrammes of retinol. Conversion to IU (International Units) is simple using this relationship:

1 microgram retinol = 3.33 IU Vitamin A.

Dietary Sources of Vitamin A

In foods vitamin A exists in two forms, preformed vitamin A and carotene, a precursor of the vitamin. Preformed vitamin A is found only in foods of animal or fish origin. The richest sources are milk, butter, cheese, egg yolk, liver and some of the fatty fish. The liver oils of fish are the richest natural sources of vitamin A, but they are used as nutritional supplements rather than foods.

Vitamin A is formed in the liver of humans and animals from a substance called carotene, so named because it was first obtained from carrots. Carotene is found in yellow and yellow-reddish fruits and vegetables such as apricots, oranges, yellow peaches, melons, carrots, squash (vegetable marrow), sweet potatoes, yams, yellow corn, pumpkin, etc. It is in green pastures and aquatic plants such as seaweed, etc. There is, however, little or no carotene in white vegetables, such as potatoes, white turnips, cauliflower, cucumber, and white onions, nor does carotene occur in any worthwhile amount in cereal or vegetable oils, excepting red palm oil which is extensively produced in West Africa and Malaysia. In Great Britain and some other countries preformed vitamin A is added to margarine to provide the same level as that in good summer butter.

The yellow colour usually present in dairy products, cheese, butter and eggs is due to carotene, but gives no indication of the amount of vitamin A present. Carotene is converted to vitamin A in the walls of the intestine and in the liver.

Losses in the Preparation of Food
Both vitamin A and carotene are stable to ordinary cooking methods, but there is some loss when butter or palm oil is used for frying. Any foods dried in the sun lose much of their vitamin potency. The main destroyer of the vitamin in fish liver oils is light, usually when they are exposed to sunlight in shop windows. Carotene is far more stable. Tinned carrots, opened more than 100 years after canning, were found to have the same carotene content as the fresh vegetables.

The Toxicity of Vitamin A and Carotene

The early explorers of the Arctic learnt from the Eskimos that it is unwise to eat the liver of the polar bear. It causes drowsiness, headache, vomiting and extensive peeling of the skin. When we consider that polar bear liver contains about 2 million IU vitamin A in 100 grams (3.5 ounces) perhaps this is not surprising.

Children and babies, however, are the main victims of vitamin A excess, usually as a result of misguided maternal enthusiasm. Intakes of between 100 000 and 500 000 IU of the vitamin give rise to loss of appetite, irritability, dry itchy skin, coarse, sparse hair and swellings over the limb bones. Death can result but if vitamin A intake is stopped soon enough, the symptoms eventually disappear. Similar symptoms were observed in adults who had taken between 45 000 and 300 000 IU of vitamin A daily over eight years for chronic skin diseases. Muscular stiffness was an added symptom in these people.

Carotene is much less toxic. Excessive intake of carrots and other carotene-rich foods can cause a yellow skin, but the condition is benign. Vitamin A is not found in toxic amounts and the skin reverts to normal colour upon ceasing the intake of carotene. Recent research suggests that, far from being toxic, a good intake of carotene is beneficial. This substance, but not vitamin A, has been found to have a protective effect against lung cancer. Cigarette smokers are advised to increase their daily carotene intake.

3

The B Complex Vitamins

Vitamin B₁ (Thiamine)

It was in 1885 that a Japanese naval surgeon, K. Takaki, demonstrated that the disease known as beri-beri, the scourge of Africa and the Far East, was associated with an excessive intake of polished rice in the diet. The disease was cured by simple dietary means by either replacing part of the rice in the rations with wheaten bread, vegetables and milk or using unpolished rice complete with husk rather than the polished variety in the diet. Parallel experiments on domestic fowls by the Dutch physician C. Eijkman showed that these birds also developed a similar disease when on polished rice diets that was cured by feeding the husk. It was not until 1926, however, that the specific 'accessory food factor' was isolated from rice polishings and the vitamin thiamine was discovered. It was designated vitamin B_1. Although vitamin B_1, or thiamine, was discovered as the result of a search for the cause of beri-beri (a disease not prevalent in Europe, USA or Australia) there is abundant evidence that much of the neuritis and other nerve troubles, indigestion, constipation, poor appetite, loss of weight, and chronic fatigue, so common in the nations mentioned, are due to a lack of thiamine.

More recently, Dr G. B. Brubacher in an international symposium on 'The Importance of Vitamins to Human Health' (1978) concluded that, 'in modern society, as a consequence of eating habits and lack of exercise, vitamin B_1 will be one of the nutrients which will become or may even be already a limiting factor in the nutrition of the general population'. A study reported in the American Journal of Clinical Nutrition in 1977 found that almost half the patients in nursing homes and elderly residents of private homes received less than two-thirds of their thiamine requirements in their diets. Evidence of a biochemical deficiency of vitamin B_1 is relatively common amongst the elderly in whom it may be associated with mental confusion. How can such deficiencies arise?

Dietary Losses of Thiamine

Thiamine is almost wholly extracted from wheat in the milling process. Hence it is removed from all refined flour products; it is virtually absent from white flour since it is present at a level of only 0.10 mg per 100 g (3.5 ounces) compared to 0.46 mg per 100 g of wholemeal flour. By law in the UK, fortification of white flour brings the level up to 0.31 mg per 100 g but this is still below that which Nature put into wheat. Refined cereals often have the thiamine removed and whilst in some cases the synthetic vitamin is added to them, it is not always the case. Such everyday dietary items as white sugar, biscuits (made from refined flour), jellies, margarine, jam, polished rice, tapioca and soft drinks contain little — or are virtually devoid of — vitamin B_1.

Many foods contain the vitamin but none has a very high concentration. The richest sources are unpolished brown rice, wheatgerm, nuts, wholegrains, wheat bran, wholemeal bread and oatflakes. Among foods of animal origin the richest amounts are found in kidney, liver, pork, lamb, chicken and fatty fish, with egg yolks supplying useful amounts. Dried brewers' yeast is the richest natural source but this is regarded as a dietary supplement rather than a basic food item.

Because thiamine is water-soluble, like other B complex vitamins, it is not stored in the body and must be taken daily to ensure good health. This vitamin is vulnerable to heat, air and water in cooking. Only a minimum of water should be used in cooking and it should first be brought to boiling point and the lid kept tightly on the saucepan to exclude air. Cooking soda partly destroys thiamine in vegetables and is never used by conscientious cooks. By far the largest losses of thiamine are due to its solubility in water, although the vitamin may be reclaimed by consumption of this water as gravy, soup, sauces, etc. Potatoes represent the only vegetable to make a significant contribution to the dietary intake of thiamine so any processing with water will leach out the vitamin. Also dipping potatoes into sulphite solution to preserve their whiteness, a process much used in the crisp and dried potato industries, neatly destroys much of the thiamine.

Function of Thiamine

The function of thiamine appears to be that of a coenzyme, namely, the conversion of blood sugar into energy. When blood sugar is utilized in the body to produce energy, pyruvic and lactic acids are formed. Thiamine is associated with enzymes which oxidize pyruvic acid and turn lactic acid into glycogen, for subsequent conversion to blood sugar.

When thiamine is deficient in the diet, these changes are incomplete. The two acids mentioned accumulate in the tissues, particularly in the brain, nerves, heart and blood. These acids irritate the tissues and retard the body's production of energy.

Wide repercussions follow. The nerve and brain cells can 'burn' only blood sugar to obtain energy. They cannot obtain their energy from fat by itself, or from protein. In more serious thiamine shortages the nerves may be damaged. Other nerve troubles are experienced, such as headaches, nerviness, neuritis, irritability, etc.

The digestive processes are also slowed down because contractions of the stomach become less vigorous, hence the food is not so effectively mixed with the digestive juices. In addition, the flow of hydrochloric acid, needed to digest proteins, slackens off or may cease altogether.

To make matters worse there are diminished secretions of bile, pancreatic and intestinal juices, all vitally necessary for a healthy digestion. Digestive enzymes, which act as ferments, are also released in smaller amounts. The net result is flatulence, gas pains, stomach trouble and poor appetite, frequently leading to loss of weight.

Constipation and Overweight

A lack of thiamine also slows down the peristaltic (wave-like) motion of the large intestine. This delays food wastes in their journey to the rectum. As a result, the faeces become hard and dry, giving rise to constipation, which may lead to the more serious condition called haemorrhoids.

It is known that overweight is often due to a shortage of thiamine. This is because starchy foods are only partially converted into energy owing to a paucity of enzymes, and tend to be stored as unwanted fat.

As less blood sugar is available for conversion to energy, the overweight person tires easily, soon becomes breathless, suffers from palpitation and generally has a craving for sweets — which are absorbed without being broken down by enzymes. Sweets give a temporary 'lift', but later on, result in a steep drop in the level of the blood sugar, causing fatigue and mental depression.

Thiamine and the Heart

Thiamine plays an important part in maintaining the health of the heart and its rhythm. Experiments with laboratory animals reveal that when thiamine is inadequate, the heart is the first organ to be affected. A thiamine deficiency initially slows down the heart beat and as this vitamin lack becomes more serious, the heart muscles, hampered by an accumulation of pyruvic and lactic acids, become irritated. This causes the heart to race and may result in heart failure. In all types of heart ailment it is prudent to ensure an adequate supply of thiamine.

In their book *The Avitaminoses*, Drs W.H. Eddy and G. Doldorf state: 'Thiamine deficiency impairs the function of the heart and increases its tendency to fluid collections.' Dr J.S. McLester, in *Nutrition and Diet in Health and Disease*, confirms the above. He says, 'a thiamine deficiency causes a degeneration of the heart muscle which are characterized by cardiac enlargement and deficient contractile power'.

There is no doubt that thiamine is essential for a healthy heart. In man, studies have revealed that the vitamin B_1 content of heart muscle from those patients dying of heart failure were lower than those who had healthy diets but had died from other causes. The conclusion was that a lifetime of inadequate thiamine intake contributed to the heart disease. This was also the conclusion of Professor Cheraskin writing in the *Journal of the American Genetics Society* (1967) who studied people throughout their lives and related their medical history to their thiamine intake. Those with the lower intakes ended up with twice the heart problems of those with higher intakes.

The Brain and Thiamine

Persons whose intake of thiamine is inadequate suffer from poor memory, lack of initiative, confused thinking and frequently from depression and fear. The reason is that the brain cells depend upon blood sugar for their energy and blood sugar, as we have remarked, cannot be transformed into energy without thiamine. Moreover, the accumulation of pyruvic and lactic acids which follows a poor supply of thiamine, has a toxic effect upon brain cells. Tests carried out by American medical scientists put this matter beyond doubt.

Conditions Where Requirements are Increased
According to most health authorities, a daily intake
of 1.5 mg of thiamine is regarded as the minimum
daily requirement for health. It is generally
accepted that during pregnancy and lactation, the
mother requires extra quantities of the order of 0.1
and 0.2 mg respectively. However, there are certain
conditions which in themselves induce less of B_1
and hence increase the need for it to maintain body
levels.

The most common is excessive consumption of
refined carbohydrates, particularly those containing
sugar and other sources of 'empty calories'. There is
a balance between carbohydrate and thiamine
intakes that is maintained in a good diet but is upset
when thiamine intakes do not keep pace with this
food constituent. Fever, surgery, infections and
other stressful conditions also call for an increased
intake of thiamine, as does increased physical
activity. Older people appear to have a greater need
for the vitamin, probably because they absorb it
from the food less efficiently.

Alcohol can exert a deleterious effect upon body
levels of thiamine and there are many medical
studies confirming this. This has now reached the
stage in the West where beri-beri has reappeared,
due solely to alcoholism, according to *The Lancet*
(1982). Heavy drinkers become thiamine deficient
not only because of low intake and losses due to
alcohol but also because they eat 'junk' foods and
consume drinks such as beer, the high carbohydrate
content of which creates a greater demand for the
vitamin.

Toxicity of Thiamine

Thiamine is perfectly safe when given orally in amounts totalling hundreds of milligrams. Occasional toxicity has been reported but only when the vitamin is given by injection.

VITAMIN B$_2$ (RIBOFLAVIN)

In 1879, a research worker named Blyth obtained from whey a substance which he named 'lactochrome', but not until 1932 was it suspected that this natural, water-soluble, yellow-green fluorescent pigment, which occurs also in plants and animals, was a most important factor in nutrition.

In 1932, Warburg and Christian isolated from yeast a yellow enzyme. Other investigators were seeking to discover the function of this enzyme in nutrition, and in 1933 it was isolated by Kuhn and his co-workers and proved to be riboflavin (vitamin B$_2$).

By 1935, Karrer and Kuhn, working separately, had successfully completed the synthesis of riboflavin.

The effect of riboflavin deficiency was noted by Stannus in 1911 when he described a group of symptoms, including sore tongue and lips, sores at the corners of the mouth and in other parts of the body, now recognized as a riboflavin deficiency. Stannus considered that these lesions were caused by dietary deficiencies, but nothing was then known of riboflavin.

Laboratory rats deprived of riboflavin developed eczema and baldness, and their eyelids became gummed and affected by conjunctivitis.

Dietary Losses of Riboflavin

Riboflavin is stable to heat under acid conditions but it is rapidly destroyed in the presence of alkalis such as cooking soda and baking powder. The great destroyer of the vitamin is light and it is known that milk in glass bottles is rapidly depleted of it by sunlight and even the strong lights of supermarkets. Packing milk in opaque cartons makes the vitamin far more stable. Even bread has been known to lose riboflavin when wrapped in clear plastic and exposed to light.

In the absence of light and alkali riboflavin is stable to most cooking methods. The greatest losses occur during cooking when the vitamin leaches out into the cooking water or into the juices when defrosting frozen foods. Utilization of the water or juices will ensure that such losses are reclaimed.

Like all the B vitamins, riboflavin is lost during the refinement and processing of foods and although it is added back in white flour and certain breakfast cereals this is not always the case. Wholefoods are thus better providers of the vitamin.

Riboflavin has a strong yellow colour and fluoresces strongly even in weak solution. It is therefore not unusual for the urine to develop a strong yellow coloration after taking the vitamin. This may be disconcerting to the individual but is in fact perfectly harmless. At least it indicates that the vitamin has been absorbed and the body is simply excreting the excess.

Sources of Riboflavin

Riboflavin is contined in milk, yeast, liver, and

leafy vegetables. It is also supplied in heart, beef muscle, veal, chicken, apricots and tomato. There is little riboflavin in cereals and legumes and in fish liver, while fish flesh contains virtually none. Beer contains significant amount of riboflavin, but an excessive intake may allow the alcohol content to have a deleterious effect upon body levels of the vitamin.

Function of Riboflavin

One function of riboflavin is to aid in utilizing carbohydrates, that is, to turn the sugars and starches we eat into energy. Riboflavin combined with protein and phosphoric acid forms enzymes needed for the breaking down of blood sugar and its conversion into energy. Riboflavin is concerned with at least five different enzymes and is essential to life. Relatively large amounts of this vitamin are stored in the liver and kidneys and a certain level is maintained in the tissues.

Riboflavin is essential for body cell respiration to ensure efficient utilization of oxygen. The vitamin is also necessary for the production and repair of body tissues and has a particular function in maintaining healthy mucous membranes, the moist surfaces of the body. Hence the eyes and mouth are usually the first to suffer in the early stages of riboflavin deficiency.

Deficiency Ailments

A dietary deficiency of riboflavin can arise from several causes, namely, faulty eating habits, food faddism of the 'I don't like salads' type, over-use of alcohol, and restricted diets for such ailments as stomach ulcers, colitis, diabetes, etc. In addition, some people do not assimilate riboflavin completely, owing to a lack of hydrochloric acid in the stomach.

According to *The Vitamins in Medicine* the following ailments can result from a shortage of riboflavin: the lips burn, become red and fissured, sometimes crusted (cheilosis); the tongue becomes inflamed, fissured and burning and there may be difficulty in swallowing; there is cracking, scaliness and softening at the corners of the mouth (stomatitis). There may be seborrheic (greasy) dermatitis, pimples and flushing of the face. The nervous symptoms include numbness, burning feet, muscular weakness, dizziness, nystagmus (rolling of the eyeballs); difficulty in walking, tremor or shaking, and mental apathy.

Eye Complaints

The eye ailments arising from a lack of riboflavin include roughness of the eyelids, watering, sensitivity to light, blurred vision, dimness of sight, conjunctivitis, burning of the eyes, twilight blindness, disorders of the cornea, retrobulbar neuritis, inflamed iris, and dilation of the pupil.

Tests have disclosed that adult laboratory animals will die on a riboflavin deficient diet and growth can be slowed or stopped in young animals. Female animals, deprived of riboflavin, may produce deformed offspring.

Avoiding Deficiency

Dietary habits are the most likely reason for a low intake of riboflavin, whether due to eating the wrong foods, poor cooking techniques, diets lacking milk and dairy products, or restricted diets taken in gastro-intestinal complaints. Alcoholism can give rise to vitamin B_2 deficiency but this is not as specific as its effect upon vitamin B_1. Amongst drugs in common use the contraceptive pill is the only one likely to lead to low body levels of riboflavin. The simplest way to overcome this problem is a daily supplement of 10 mg.

Therapeutic Uses of Riboflavin

Recurrent mouth ulcers have been claimed to be prevented by daily intakes of 20 mg or more of vitamin B_2. Similar trials on stomach and duodenal ulcers did not give such a dramatic response but this is because these lesions are the result of factors besides riboflavin deficiency.

Ulceration of the cornea of the eye will sometimes respond to high potency supplementation with vitamin B_2. In a study of 47 patients suffering from eye and eyesight problems, six of whom were affected by cataracts, reported in *Prevention* (1970), a high rate of remission was claimed with riboflavin but only while the high intakes of the vitamin were maintained. Such results confirmed similar studies on animals suffering from various eye conditions, but responses were better when the whole of the vitamin B complex was used therapeutically.

Toxicity of Riboflavin

Riboflavin is virtually non-toxic. It is so safe that it is accepted as a natural colouring agent that may be added to foods.

Vitamin B₃ (Niacin)

Niacin, known variously as niacinamide, nicotinic acid, and nicotinamide, was discovered by Huber in 1867, but its significance in nutrition was not realized until 1938 when Kuhn and Vetter isolated it from heart muscle and Frost and Elvehjein discovered that it had growth-stimulating properties.

Niacin occurs in all living cells. It forms part of the body's enzyme system and promotes oxidative processes and the transport of hydrogen atoms.

For the last two centuries, the disease known as pellagra, from *pelle agra*, meaning rough skin, has occurred fairly constantly in districts where maize is the staple item of food.

It is now known that maize is deficient in tryptophane, an essential amino acid which is a precursor of niacin. The conversion of tryptophane to niacin is considered to occur in the tissues, not as a result of the action of intestinal micro-organisms.

Niacin is present in almost all the tissues, chiefly as a coenzyme, and more is contained in the liver than any other organ. Chronic alcoholics and those with serious liver ailments, may have difficulty in storing niacin because of this fact.

Niacin is resistant to the oxygen in the air and also to the heat of cooking but, like riboflavin, it is easily leached away in the water used for cooking.

Sources of Niacin

The amount of niacin in foods available as a vitamin is determined by three factors:

1   the level of the free vitamin;

2   the quantity of the bound vitamin, and
3   the amount that is derived within the body from the essential amino acid L-tryptophane in the diet.

This amino acid is needed for other functions besides acting as a precursor of nicotinic acid but the accepted conversion rate is that 60 mg tryptophane will give rise to 1 mg nicotinic acid. In wheat flour, for example, as much as 77 per cent of the niacin is in the bound form (known as niacytin) and the free vitamin is not liberated completely unless the flour is baked under alkaline conditions. When bound, nicotinic acid is completely unavailable to the body. Fortunately nicotinic acid is very stable to all conditions of cooking and the main losses, like those of the other B vitamins, are due to leaching into water and meat drippings. Hence as long as these liquids are consumed in one way or another you can obtain the full benefits of the vitamin.

Rich sources of nicotinic acid include lean meats, wheatgerm, organ meats, fish, yeast and yeast extracts and some wholegrains. Cereals provide moderate quantities of the vitamin but some of this is in the bound form. Instant coffee, whether decaffeinated or not, is a good source of nicotinic acid. Vegetables, green and root, and dairy products do not provide much of the vitamin.

In terms of weight, the daily requirements of nicotinic acid are amounts for adults of 18 mg for men and 15 mg for women. During pregnancy and lactation a woman needs an additional 3 mg and 6 mg respectively. Growing children need from 10 mg to 19 mg daily, depending upon age.

Pellagra

Gross deficiency of niacin causes the disease known as pellagra, which affects the skin, intestinal tract and nervous system. A comprehensive study of pellagra was made in 1725 by the physician Don Gaspal Casal in the province of Asturias, Spain, where this disease was first recognized. Further studies were made when it later occurred in the Austrian Tyrol and Rumania, where the people lived on diets containing almost no flesh foods or cheese.

Towards the close of the nineteenth century, the connection between pellagra and an inadequate diet was obscured by the development of the new science of microbiology, because there was then a tendency to ascribe every disease of unknown cause to the action of a micro-organism. This view was shared by the eminent Italian scientist Lombroso, and valuable research time was lost.

Search for its Cause

In the USA Dr Joseph Goldberger, who in 1915 was investigating pellagra for the Public Health Department, noticed that in three public hospitals in the Southern states, the disease did not spread from patients to staffs despite the absence of any special precautions. He also observed that the hospital staffs had a more varied diet than the inmates, because staff members supplemented hospital fare with food from outside, a privilege denied to patients.

Goldberger became convinced that pellagra could

not be a communicable disease, but was due to the hospitals' inadequate dietary, mostly cereals. He therefore requested that a supply of meat, tinned salmon, eggs, etc., be made to the inmates, and after this improved diet pellagra was eliminated from these institutions.

It is now recognized that economic conditions influence the food supply and provide conditions for the development of pellagra, as this ailment rarely occurs among those who enjoy a varied diet, including ample protein. Pellagra mostly affects poor people, who have to exist on a limited choice of foods, lacking protein.

Other Niacin Deficiency Ailments

In a mild deficiency of niacin the tongue is usually a bright red at the tip, but further back, it is coated. A furred tongue and bad breath often indicate a lack of niacin. When canker sores and small ulcers form on the cheeks or under the tongue there is every likelihood that the niacin intake is inadequate.

A mild lack of niacin causes digestive disturbances, because the secretion of hydrochloric acid in the stomach falls away and stomach trouble follows. As this acid is required to promote the assimilation of protein, iron and calcium, anaemia and nerve disorders can result.

With the digestive system disorganized food is not properly absorbed, causing flatulence, constipation or diarrhoea. Gradually the entire intestinal tract becomes inflamed, to be felt noticeably in the region of the rectum and anus. Unless this condition is rectified, it may lead to colitis.

A deficiency of niacin can also cause dizziness,

insomnia, irritability, nausea, vomiting and recurring headaches. In more severe deficiencies, there is a sensation of strain and tension with deep depression, which may cause the sufferer either to cry or feel like crying.

The most likely cause of low body levels of niacin is a poor diet that is low in the free vitamin contains excessive amounts of cereals that have a high percentage of bound niacin and has a low protein content supplying little tryptophane. Alcoholism can also lead to nicotinic acid deficiency both through poor diet associated with the condition and the direct effect of alcohol on the absorption and utilization of the vitamin. Deficiency of nicotinic acid can be induced by the use of sulphanamide drugs and by other antibiotics like penicillin. Such drugs tend to cause deficiency of the B complex as a whole, but drugs such as those based on mercaptopurine, used in the treatment of leukaemia, produce a specific deficiency of nicotinic acid. It is generally recognized that a daily supplement of 50 mg of the vitamin is sufficient to overcome deficiencies induced by drip and alcohol.

Therapeutic Uses of Niacin

Niacin in the form of nicotinic acid and nicotinamide (niacinamide) has been used with some success in treating a variety of conditions. Some of these are now summarized.

Schizophrenia

The mental symptoms associated with pellagra are similar to those seen in schizophrenia and include tension, depression, personality problems and mental fatigue. These observations led Drs H. Oswald and A. Hoffer of the University of Saskatchewan in Canada to treat schizophrenic patients with high doses (between 3 and 6 grams daily) of nicotinic acid. The results were successful enough to stimulate other doctors to try the treatment on their patients and Dr D. Hawkins has treated over 4000 schizophrenics successfully in his New York clinic. Sometimes the success rate is higher if other vitamins like C and B_6 are given at the same time. However, not all trials using high potency nicotinic acid were successful and for this reason such treatment is best left in the hands of qualified practitioners. Where the vitamin's therapy is more likely to help, however, is in treating schizophrenic children. A daily dose of 3 grams plus 300 mg vitamin C and 200 mg vitamin B_6 was found to be of value by Dr A. Hoffer. Children with poor learning ability are often helped by lower intakes of 1 — 2 g of nicotinic acid daily plus vitamin C (200 mg) and vitamin B_6 (200 mg).

Alcoholism
Alcoholics often show mental symptoms similar to those of schizophrenics and are treated in a comparable fashion. Both nicotinic acid and nicotinamide have been used, the latter because it is better tolerated at the high doses needed. On intakes of up to 6 g daily, Dr R.F. Smith of Michigan reported benefit in over 430 of 500 alcoholics treated. Not only did the symptoms improve but many of the individuals were cured of their alcohol habits.

Reducing Blood Cholesterol Levels
Nicotinic acid but not nicotinamide will reduce blood cholesterol levels. High doses are required and the most consistent results were obtained by taking 1 g nicotinic acid after each meal. This is best carried out by starting with 100 mg after each meal and gradually building the dose up to 1000 mg after each meal over a period of fourteen days or so. This treatment decreases blood cholesterol levels by an average of 26 per cent after one year's therapy but the nicotinic acid must be taken continuously to maintain the lower level.

Toxicity of Niacin and Niacinamide

Nicotinic acid causes the blood vessels to dilate when given at high levels so flushing of the face, a sensation of heat and headache may occur in some people. The symptoms are transient but can be distressing. Although these effects are not noted to the same extent with niacinamide (nicotinamide), this form of the vitamin can cause depression in high doses. High doses of all forms of the vitamin should be avoided during pregnancy, particularly during the first 56 days.

Occasionally nicotinic acid will cause dry skin, rashes, itching and boils. Abdominal cramps, diarrhoea and nausea sometimes occur, but only with high doses of the vitamin. Hence nicotinic acid should not be taken at high levels by those suffering from gastric and duodenal ulcers. All side-effects disappear on ceasing to take the vitamin, so there is no permanent damage.

Vitamin B₆ (Pyridoxine)

In 1934, Gyorgyi reported having discovered a nutritional factor (distinct from the water- soluble factors then known), a lack of which caused a particular type of dermatitis in rats, somewhat resembling pink disease in infants. This new factor was called vitamin B_6 and was isolated in 1939 by several different investigators. In the same year, the vitamin was synthesized by Kuhn in Germany, and by Harris and Folkers in America.

Sources of Pyridoxine

Pyridoxine is widely distributed in foods of all kinds and is particularly rich in liver, kidney, pork, ham and veal amongst the meats; fresh fish; bananas, avocados, prunes, raisins; peas, beans, lentils, unpolished rice; peanuts, walnuts and wholegrain cereals. Milk and vegetables are relatively poor sources of the vitamin.

In food, vitamin B_6 exists in three forms known as pyridoxine, pyridoxal and pyridoxamine. All three are equally acceptable to the human body as vitamins and are converted after absorption into the biologically active coenzyme known as pyridoxine-50-phosphate.

All three forms of vitamin B_6 appear to be stable to most cooking methods. None are affected by acids, alkalis or oxidation, so the main losses tend to be due to leaching out into the cooking water. Considerable destruction of the vitamin can occur in milk subjected to high temperature. This is due less to the heat than to interaction with other milk components. Until this was realized, it was not uncommon for babies fed such milk to develop convulsions due to lack of the vitamin. Modern methods of milk drying have now overcome this problem.

What Experiments Revealed

Experiments with laboratory animals have revealed that skin lesions, anaemia, cardiovascular ailments, fatty degeneration of the liver, kidney trouble and nerve lesions have resulted when the animals were kept on diets deficient in vitamin B_6.

Dr H.H. Schroeder of the Department of Internal Medicine, Washington University School of Medicine, St Louis, USA, states that too little pyridoxine in the diet of experimental monkeys produced hardening of the arteries and a deficiency of this vitamin in rats caused high blood pressure.

It was noted in some instances that the antibody formation in test animals was defective and that there was increased susceptibility to infection, for example, pneumonia. In human beings lack of the vitamin can give rise to nervous problems, mental depression and convulsions, particularly in infants. Other signs of deficiency include skin complaints, sore tongue and a particular type of anaemia that is cured only by vitamin B_6 treatment.

Function of Pyridoxine

Pyridoxine is involved, as a coenzyme, in more than sixty enzymic reactions within the body. Many of these are concerned with the metabolism of the amino acids supplied by the protein we eat. Some of these amino acids in turn are precursors of substances that are essential for nerve and brain functions. Therefore it is not surprising that lack of the vitamin gives rise to nerve problems.

One of these essential amino acids is called L-tryptophane. Under the influence of pyridoxine this is converted to the B vitamin nicotinic acid. It is also converted to a substance known as serotonin which is essential for nerve and brain function and whose lack produces depression.

Another amino acid is called L-glutamic acid which requires vitamin B_6 for its conversion to gamma-aminobutyric acid (GABA) — a natural calming agent for the central nervous system. Deficiency of the vitamin means that GABA is not produced and convulsions can result.

The third specific amino acid that undergoes transformation with the aid of pyridoxine is L-methionine. The first product of its metabolism is homocysteine which is a toxic compound. Usually this material exists only transitorily and is immediately converted to non-toxic compounds. This change is dependent upon vitamin B_6, so in its absence the toxic homocysteine builds up. The result of this is rapid development of atherosclerosis, i.e. fatty deposits in blood vessels. Hence one factor that protects against this complaint is an adequate intake of vitamin B_6. We can assume therefore that the vitamin is also concerned in fat metabolism.

Pyridoxine and Human Ailments

With our increasing knowledge about how pyridoxine functions in the body it is becoming apparent that when these functions go wrong the cause can often be related either to a deficiency of the vitamin in the diet or an increased requirement induced by disease or by medicinal drugs. We shall therefore look at how therapeutic intakes of the vitamin have conferred benefit in certain complaints.

Depression Caused by the Contraceptive Pill

In various studies a high proportion of women using the contraceptive pill were found to exhibit abnormal metabolism of tryptophane. One result of this is a high incidence of mild depression. The reason for this in some cases (19 out of 39 in one study) was a deficiency of vitamin B_6 caused by the synthetic oestrogen present in the pill. All of these nineteen women were cured of their depression symptoms simply by taking 40 mg or so of the vitamin daily. Those showing no signs of B_6 deficiency in their blood did not respond to the vitamin, presumably because their depression had other causes.

Premenstrual Syndrome (PMS)

The main premenstrual syndrome symptoms are depression, irritability, tiredness, breast discomfort, swollen abdomen and puffy fingers and ankles. Treatment with 100 mg per day of vitamin B_6 from day 10 of one cycle to day 3 of the next or simply taking 50 mg of the vitamin daily caused an overall improvement in all the symptoms in 63 per cent of the women. More than 80 per cent of those treated were cured of premenstrual headache, the most common symptom noted. The reason that vitamin B_6 helps in this condition is that some women appear to have a greater requirement for pyridoxine in the days just before their period commences.

Bronchial Asthma

Vitamin B_6 has been referred to as the anti-allergy vitamin on account of its successful use in treating some allergic skin diseases, in hay fever and in bronchial asthma. A dose of 100 mg twice daily has helped clear up symptoms in asthmatic children in studies carried out in the USA. It took a month for the treatment to take effect but improvement was continued and it was possible for conventional drugs to be gradually phased out since these are palliative rather than curative.

Kidney Stones

Most kidney stones are due to an upset in calcium metabolism whereby it is deposited in the kidneys, causing the build-up of stones. It was reported in the *American Journal of Clinical Nutrition* that a high intake of the mineral magnesium (300 mg daily) plus 25 mg of vitamin B_6 per day can repress the deposition of calcium and hence reduce the possibility of kidney stone formation. Vitamin B_6 helps particularly by reducing the formation of oxalic acid which is the precipitating agent for calcium.

Toxicity of Vitamin B_6

The vitamin is remarkably non-toxic. None of the people involved in the various trials mentioned above complained of side-effects. The only condition where pyridoxine is contra-indicated is in those people who suffer from Parkinson's disease and are being treated with the drug levo-dopa.

Probable Requirement

The probable human requirement of pyridoxine is

considered to range from 2 to 3 mg daily. However, as we have seen, requirements can increase in some people and in certain conditions.

VITAMIN B_{12} (CYANOCOBALAMIN)

In 1926, Minot and Murphy showed that raw liver is curative in cases of pernicious anaemia. Other research workers began to use liver concentrates instead of liver, and in 1948 it was announced both by Lester Smith in England and Rickes in America that they had isolated the anti-pernicious anaemia factor in pure crystalline form. It was named vitamin B_{12}, and cobalt is an essential constituent of the molecule.

The Intrinsic Factor

In 1929, Castle showed that beef muscle or beef liver, when mixed with normal gastric juice and administered to patients suffering from pernicious anaemia, restored normal blood formation. He therefore suggested that there were two factors necessary to prevent pernicious anaemia. One was the intrinsic factor present in normal gastric juice; the other was the extrinsic factor present in food. Those suffering from pernicious anaemia lacked the intrinsic factor so that they were unable to absorb the extrinsic factor. This was eventually proved to be vitamin B_{12}. Hence their deficiency of the vitamin was caused not by lack of it in the diet but the inability to assimilate it. Once the absorption system was bypassed by injecting the vitamin, their pernicious anaemia was cured. Usually 1 milligram every month given by intra-muscular injection is sufficient to control the anaemia.

Other factors that contribute to lack of absorption of vitamin B_{12} are a lack of hydrochloric acid in the stomach (achlorhydria) and a shortage of calcium in the intestinal digestive juices. Tapeworms in the intestine can claim the vitamin before it can be absorbed so a deficiency is produced. Similarly an abnormal number and type of intestinal bacteria can use up the vitamin B_{12} in the food and make it unavailable to the body.

The Effects of Vitamin B_{12} Deficiency

Despite the tiny amounts of vitamin B_{12} necessary to maintain health it is probably required by every cell of the body and its deficiency is most severely felt in those tissues with a rapid turnover. These are in the blood-forming organs and in the lining of the gastro-intestinal tract, hence the anaemia and the effect on the digestive organs seen in vitamin B_{12} deficiency. The most insidious effect of deficiency, however, is on the nervous system where the nerve fibres degenerate in the spinal cord and elsewhere. Once the nervous system is affected, a stage is reached where degeneration becomes irreversible, even on treatment with the vitamin. The blood normalizes but the nerves do not.

In addition to symptoms in the blood and nervous system, vitamin B_{12} deficiency gives rise to a smooth, sore tongue, menstrual disorders, listlessness, tremors and excessive pigmentation that affects only coloured people.

Function of Vitamin B_{12}

Vitamin B_{12} is essential to maintain the myelin sheath of nerves. Myelin may be regarded as performing the same function for nerve fibres that insulation does to electric cables. Lack of the vitamin causes breaks in the myelin sheath, so short-circuiting the nerve impulses that travel along the nerve fibre. Pernicious anaemia injures the nerve cells, especially those in the spinal cord. This damage results in a jerky gait, a swaying of the body, lack of co-ordination and loss of balance.

In the formation of blood, vitamin B_{12} works hand-in-hand with folic acid. Both vitamins are required for the synthesis of the constituents of deoxyribonucleic acid (DNA) which is the very basis of body and blood cell production. In the absence of either or both vitamins, blood cell production grinds to a halt and pernicious anaemia results.

Sources of Vitamin B_{12}

Meaningful sources of vitamin B_{12} are confined to foods of animal origin. Organ meats such as liver and kidney contain the highest concentration of the vitamin, but muscle meat provides useful quantities. All types of fish are good sources of B_{12} and dairy products contain sufficient quantities to provide daily requirements. For this reason lacto-vegetarians should obtain ample supplies from dairy products. Fortunately the vitamin is stable to all cooking methods because in meats and dairy products it is attached to proteins. Vegans, however, should be aware of possible deficiencies of the vitamin because of their dietary habits. There is no evidence that vegans are more likely to suffer from pernicious anaemia (gross deficiency) than non-vegans, but they invariably have lower blood concentrations of vitamin B_{12} and probably exist on sub-optimal levels.

Therapeutic Uses of Vitamin B_{12}

Vitamin B_{12} is used in treating pernicious anaemia and this disease will not respond to anything else.

Old people with mild mental problems will often respond to the vitamin. Those who exhibited mental apathy, moodiness, poor memory, paranoia and confusion have benefited from vitamin B_{12} therapy. However it must be realized that the absorption of the vitamin from the gastro-intestinal tract is very limited, because of the unique intrinsic factor mechanism, and the only way to obtain large intakes is by intra-muscular injection.

Dr H. Grabner, in an article in the *Munich Medical Weekly*, reported the following ailments as responding well to vitamin B_{12}: ulcers, rheumatic diseases and muscular dystrophy. Other ailments that have benefited from this vitamin are bursitis, migraine, shingles and psoriasis.

According to the *Journal of the American Medical Association*, vitamin B_{12} is used successfully for hepatitis (inflammation of the liver). Other reports advise of the beneficial use of vitamin B_{12} for asthma, osteoarthritis and osteoporosis (porous bones).

There is little doubt, too, that the vitamin B_{12} can help in the relief of muscle fatigue and in supplying extra energy. Appetite, mood, energy and sleep quality were all improved with vitamin B_{12} and there was also an overall feeling of well-being.

One effect of the components of the contraceptive pill is to reduce vitamin B_{12} levels and it can be beneficial to increase the intake when taking this pill. During pregnancy and lactation, requirements increase mainly due to the demands of the foetus in the former case, since any rapidly growing tissues like this need ample vitamin B_{12}. Extra intake from the food or supplements are generally recommended in all these conditions.

Daily Requirements

Apart from vegans and some vegetarians it is highly likely that anyone partaking of meat, fish and dairy products is going to obtain at least 4 micrograms in the diet. Absorption of as little as one microgram daily is probably sufficient to prevent deficiency. Unlike the other B vitamins, there is significant storage of vitamin B_{12} in the liver and since daily requirements are so small it takes some time for gross deficiency symptoms to appear if absorption of it from the food stops. This can be anything from six months to two years but during the period of depletion body levels of B_{12} are, of course, suboptimal.

Toxicity of Vitamin B_{12}

Vitamin B_{12} is virtually non-toxic at any dose. Very rarely a reaction has followed injections of the vitamin but there are no reports of any adverse reactions when it is taken by orally.

FOLIC ACID

Dr Mary Wills in 1931 was studying pregnant women in India when she noted that they were prone to a particular type of anaemia that did not respond to iron, to the known vitamins nor to liver extracts. As the diet of the women was composed mainly of polished rice and white bread it was clear that some dietary factor was missing. It was not until ten years later, however, that this factor was discovered.

The compounds known collectively as folic acid were discovered in 1941 by Mitchell, Snell and Williams after research work on a concentrate obtained from spinach. Subsequently, this factor was obtained from liver.

In 1944 these research workers obtained concentrated folic acid in a high degree of potency from spinach, namely, 137 000 times as active as the original product. By 1945, the successful synthesis and chemical identification of folic acid was accomplished by a group of scientists working in the Lederle Laboratories, USA.

Sources of Supply

Folic acid derived its name from the word 'foliage' and this vitamin is supplied in fresh, deep-green, leafy vegetables. Liver and kidney are also rich sources of supply. Beef and wheatgerm contain some folic acid, but root vegetables, pork, ham, lamb, cheese, milk, corn, rice and many tinned foods are very poor sources of folic acid.

One complication in assessing the folic acid content of food is the fact that there are many types of folic acid present, not all of which are utilized as the vitamin. For example, as little as 30 per cent of folic acid in some foods and as much as 75 per cent in others actually function as a vitamin. Supplements have the advantage that they are 100 per cent available as the vitamin folic acid.

Cooking vegetables in large volumes of water causes leaching out of the folic acid, and the rule is to boil them in the minimum amount of water or to pressure cook them. The vitamin is very unstable to oxygen at high temperatures, but vitamin C helps to protect the folic acid and both are usually present together in vegetables anyway. Light destroys folic acid and the destruction is catalysed by the other B vitamin riboflavin; hence, taken overall, as much as 45 per cent of folic acid can be lost during the processing and cooking of vegetables, fruits and dairy products. Eating fruits and vegetables raw helps preserve the folic acid content. It is probably this combined with their high intake of such foods that ensures that vegetarians and vegans are usually replete with the vitamin.

Dietary Considerations

A poor diet combined with the destructive cooking methods referred to above lead to nutritional folic acid deficiency in all age groups. In the USA, for example, studies on school children indicated that many had an intake just one-fifth of that believed necessary for health. At the other end of the scale, many studies in the USA and Europe found that elderly people tend to suffer from folic acid deficiency due mainly to poor diets but also less efficient absorption of the vitamin from their digestive systems. As much as 67 per cent of old people may be folic acid deficient in the UK, some to such an extent as to show signs of gross deficiency.

One of the largest population groups prone to folic acid deficiency world-wide is pregnant females. The World Health Organization has estimated that between one-third and one-half of all pregnant females are deficient during the last three months of pregnancy. Requirements during pregnancy are likely double those at other times, the reason being that the foetus is a rapidly growing body and needs adequate supplies from its mother who herself may then become deficient. In Western countries supplementation with folic acid is becoming accepted as the norm during pregnancy.

Deficiency Ailments

A deficiency of folic acid can give rise to any of the following ailments: anaemia, diarrhoea, glossitis, (inflammation of the tongue), gastro-intestinal disorders, lack of hydrochloric acid in the stomach, and a decrease in the normal number of white blood corpuscles. Folic acid has been used with success in the treatment of anaemia associated with rheumatoid arthritis, in coeliac disease (a chronic intestinal disorder of infants and children) and in disorders arising from the use of sulpha drugs.

The main manifestation of lack of folic acid is megaloblastic anaemia. In this condition the red blood cells become very large and uneven in size and shape with a shorter life span than round red blood cells. The outward signs of deficiency are similar to those associated with other types of anaemia. These include weakness, fatigue, irritability, sleeplessness, culminating in mild mental symptoms such as confusion and forgetfulness.

Function of Folic Acid

Folic acid is essential to the metabolism of the

nucleic acids which are of two types: ribonucleic acids (RNA) and deoxyribonucleic acid (DNA). These acids play a central role in protein synthesis, a function that is absolutely essential to life processes. Hence we can sum up the main role of folic acid as being necessary to make cells divide and multiply, particularly those of the blood which have a fast turnover. We have seen that vitamin B_{12} is also concerned with DNA synthesis and in processes like red blood cell production and body cell turnover the two vitamins are inextricably linked.

It is a fact that the megaloblastic anaemia produced by vitamin B_{12} deficiency can be cleared up with massive doses of folic acid. However, what folic acid cannot do is to cure the nervous degeneration that is the result of vitamin B_{12} deficiency. It is therefore vitally important that once megaloblastic anaemia has been discovered the vitamin deficiency should be determined, i.e. either folic acid or vitamin B_{12}. Failure to diagnose vitamin B_{12} deficiency or treat it incorrectly will cause irreversible nerve degeneration.

Therapeutic Uses of Folic Acid

Resistance to Disease

One result of reduced folic acid in the body is a lowered resistance to disease. This is particularly serious in new-born babies who are born to folic acid deficient mothers, since the initial build-up of resistance after birth is dependent upon the vitamin amongst other factors. Adults, too, can help ward off illness with an adequate intake of folic acid. Sometimes people with recurring infections are unable to absorb the vitamin and they can be treated only by injecting large doses of folic acid.

Brain Function

Reports in the *New England Journal of Medicine* (1975) stated that mentally disturbed and retarded people will sometimes respond favourably to folic acid treatment. Schizophrenia and other mental conditions will also be helped in some people by high potency intakes of folic acid, according to reports from Northwick Park Hospital, Middlesex. Doses range from 5 mg to 20 mg daily, but because of present legislation they can only be administered under medical supervision.

Daily Requirements

Although there is no complete agreement among official bodies regarding the folic acid requirements required for health, a rough average is 300 to 500 microgrammes. This should be doubled during pregnancy and breast-feeding. As a typical, mixed, Western diet provides between 150 and 300 microgrammes folic acid daily, it would appear that many people are on the borderline of deficiency.

Toxicity of Folic Acid

The vitamin is usually well tolerated when taken orally. Occasionally there have been reports of loss of appetite, nausea, flatulence and abdominal distension when the vitamin is taken at the level of 15 mg per day. Sleep disturbance and irritability may also occur, while some people become overactive with high intakes of folic acid.

Para-Aminobenzoic Acid (PABA)

PABA was first synthesized by Fischer in 1863, but it was only admitted to the B complex family in 1940, after research work by Ansbacher. Later, Prof. D. D. Woods at Oxford University had observed that PABA was essential to the growth of bacteria. He proved that sulphanamide drugs exerted their anti-infective action because, being similar in structure to PABA, they attached themselves to the enzymes in bacteria that usually combined with PABA. In so doing, they denied the bacteria access to the PABA that they needed to thrive. Hence this competitive antagonism explained the antibiotic function of the sulphanamides.

Although PABA is undoubtedly a vitamin for micro-organisms there is no hard evidence that it is one for man. What is established is that PABA is present as part of the complex chemical structure of the B vitamin folic acid. It must be stressed that this does not mean that the body is able to convert PABA into folic acid. It is now apparent, from modern research, that PABA does have some functions within the body and can confer benefit in some animal conditions.

PABA in Animals

In animal experiments there is evidence that PABA is essential in the production of body protein. In addition it appears to be a necessary factor for the normal synthesis of red blood cells. Both of these functions in animals are most likely manifested through PABA as an intermediate for folic acid rather than a vitamin in its own right. There is no doubt, however, that a sign of PABA deficiency in animals is premature greying of the hair. Supplementing the diet with the factor restores the hair colour to normal. Occasionally PABA has restored the natural hair colour to human beings when given orally, but the success rate is below that for animals. This is probably because PABA represents only one factor among many required to maintain a normal-coloured and healthy head of hair.

PABA in Man

The only proved beneficial effect of PABA in man relates to its action on the skin. One particular complaint is vitiligo which has defied conventional medical treatment for years. Vitiligo is characterized by the sudden appearance of light areas on the skin, particularly those places exposed to sunlight. The normal production of the skin pigment melanin appears to have stopped in these areas. The condition causes no symptoms apart from the skin discoloration so the problem is cosmetic rather than clinical.

Treatment with PABA consists of injecting the material and taking it orally up to a total daily intake of 200 to 300 mg daily. Sometimes oral administration is sufficient. After two weeks, new light-coloured pigmentation often appears in the affected areas although six to eight months' treatment will probably be required before full colouring is restored. In addition, the B vitamins pyridoxine and pantothenic acid appear to complement the action of PABA as well as adequate intakes of the minerals zinc and manganese.

PABA as a Sunscreen Agent

The most successful use of PABA in man is as a sunscreen agent applied to the skin. In comparative clinical trials, PABA as a sunscreen lotion was the best protective against sunburn. The most effective solution turned out to be a 5 per cent concentration of PABA in aqueous alcohol and there are several proprietary sunscreen lotions based upon this. Oral PABA combined with the tropical product ensure two-pronged protection against the sun by ensuring there is no body deficiency.

Recent experiments on mice carried out at the University of Miami, USA, have indicated that PABA appears to protect these animals against skin cancer induced by ultraviolet light. A similar protective action of PABA against human skin cancer is possible, according to these researchers, so it is a wise precaution for fair-skinned people to protect their skin with this factor when exposed to strong sun.

Food Sources of PABA

PABA occurs in foodstuffs as a component of the B complex, so the richest sources of it are liver, eggs, molasses, wholegrains, brewers' yeast and wheatgerm. The concentration is not high — yeasts vary from 0.5 to 10 mg PABA per 100 grams, depending on the type of yeast — but its wide distribution ensures a daily intake of 10 mg or so from a good diet. No one knows the daily requirement of PABA, so it is impossible to determine whether or not this is sufficient for health.

PABA is a stable substance, so losses in food cooking are more likely to come from leaching into cooking fluids rather than by destruction. Food processing and refining are likely to cause wholesale loss, as with other members of the B complex.

Toxicity of PABA

PABA is usually tolerated in low doses, but high intakes can give rise to nausea, vomiting, itch, rash and liver damage, especially on prolonged treatment. The only contra-indication is for those taking sulphanamide as antibiotics.

PANTOTHENIC ACID (VITAMIN B5)

The name pantothenic acid is derived from the Greek work *panthos* which means 'everywhere', a name chosen because the vitamin is universally distributed in food and in all living matter. It was discovered as a result of research into a certain type of dermatitis found only around the eyes and beaks of chicks. The known B vitamins at the time — riboflavin, nicotinic acid and pyridoxine — had no effect upon the disease, but it could be cured with yeast and other foods rich in B vitamins. Fortunately a strain of yeast was developed that needed the new factor in order to grow, so this ready-made assay system enabled it to be studied. The net result was the isolation of a new vitamin, pantothenic acid, by Dr R. J. Williams of the University of Texas, from rice husks. This discovery in 1939 was followed a year later by its synthesis in Germany, Switzerland and America.

The Function of Pantothenic Acid

In rats, pantothenic acid has the ability to prevent greying of black hair. It has had the same effect occasionally in people but, like PABA, a greater rate of success is achieved when other factors are taken at the same time.

In man, and probably in other species, pantothenic acid is a constituent of coenzyme A which is essential for energy production, for fat and cholesterol metabolism, for antibody formation and to ensure a healthy nervous system. Its involvement with cholesterol is particularly important since this compound is the starting material for production of anti-stress hormones by the body. Pantothenic acid is necessary to convert cholesterol into these essential body constituents, hence its description as the anti-stress vitamin.

Deficiency Symptoms
There are no specific deficiency symptoms in man apart from the 'burning feet' syndrome. The earliest symptoms are arching, burning or throbbing pains in the feet. These discomforts become more intense and develop eventually into sharp, stabbing, shooting pains that may spread as far as the knee, causing agonizing pain. The complaint is associated with poor diet and responds only to pantothenic acid treatment. Other more generalized symptoms of deficiency include insomnia, fatigue and depression. Alcoholics are particularly prone to nervous disease and psychosis that may be related to pantothenic acid deficiency, although it must be remembered that these people tend to have an overall deficiency of the whole vitamin B complex.

Dietary Loss of Pantothenic Acid
Although the vitamin is widely distributed in

nature, substantial losses can occur during the dry-processing of foods. The processing of wheat grains to white flour results in wholesale destruction and loss of the vitamin. Domestic cooking and baking cause little loss of the vitamin but roasting of meat destroys 40 per cent of the vitamin content. It is water-soluble, so losses of pantothenic acid into cooking water and into the thawed drippings from frozen foods can be considerable. Acid and alkaline conditions during cooking are particularly destructive to the vitamin, so care should be taken when using cooking acids like vinegar and sodium bicarbonate.

Occurrence in Foods and Requirements

The largest concentrations of pantothenic acid are found in meat, poultry, fish, wholegrain cereals and nuts. Less rich sources are fruit, vegetables and milk. When isolated from natural foods, pantothenic acid is an unstable, pale-yellow, oily liquid that is soluble in water. For this reason the vitamin is incorporated into dietary supplements as calcium pantothenate, a white, stable, crystalline product that is just as active as the natural pantothenic acid.

The human requirements for pantothenic acid are thought to be about 10 milligrams daily but this must be considered an absolute minimum. There is increased requirement for the vitamin during any stress situation, after an injury and following antibiotic therapy. The intestinal bacteria that inhabit the lower end of the intestine synthesize the vitamin and it is quite likely that the body can utilize this, but the total amount provided by this route is uncertain. Nevertheless, it is a sound idea and beneficial to take supplements of pantothenic acid whilst on antibiotic therapy, since these drugs are likely to destroy the 'friendly' bacteria also.

Therapeutic Activity of Pantothenic Acid

Resistance to Infection

One aspect of pantothenic acid deficiency in animals and man is a lowered resistance to disease. The reason is that this vitamin along with vitamin B_6 is essential in the production of antibodies, those factors necessary to destroy harmful bacteria and viruses, hence increased intake during infections can be beneficial.

Allergy

Studies reported from Hungary claimed that children with allergic skin reactions were relieved of the problem by simply taking 100 mg of pantothenic acid daily. In the USA respiratory problems induced by allergic reactions were cleared up in adults by taking 100 mg of the vitamin at night. Excess mucus secretion during sleep was reduced considerably on this treatment so that the people taking the vitamin woke up refreshed and without the cough and stuffed-up feeling that were features before treatment.

Arthritis

One feature of pantothenic acid deficiency noted in animal experiments was the development of an arthritic condition. Further studies indicated that people suffering from arthritis usually had lower blood levels of pantothenic acid than those who did not suffer from the disease. These results, along with other observations, were sufficient to encourage doctors in Great Britain to try pantothenic acid (in the form of calcium pantothenate) in treating arthritis. The results published in 1980 were highly promising: the duration of morning stiffness, the degree of disability and the severity of pain were all reduced by the action of pantothenic acid alone. Benefit is far more likely in rheumatoid arthritis than in osteoarthritis and there is a high rate of success in the former. The dosage required is 500 mg (one tablet) daily for two days; 1000 mg (2 tablets) for three days; 1500 mg (3 tablets) for four days and finally 2000 mg (4 tablets) per day thereafter for a period of two months. Once relief is obtained the dosage can be reduced to that needed to maintain this relief.

Toxicity of Pantothenic Acid

There is no evidence that pantothenic acid is toxic in any quantity, even at the high doses taken in the arthritis studies.

BIOTIN

The discovery of biotin was due to a casual observation by Bateman in 1916 that a high concentration of egg white in experimental diets is toxic.

Subsequently, it was found that certain foods, which include liver and yeast, contain an organic substance that protects test rats against the toxic effects of 'egg white' injury.

Between 1913 and 1940 this organic substance was the subject of intensive study by Gyorgyi and co-workers. By 1936 a crystalline substance had been obtained from egg *yolk* and named biotin. From about a quarter of a ton of dried egg yolk, one milligram of active biotin was obtained.

In 1940 biotin was isolated from liver and its structure established. The synthesis of this vitamin was effected in 1943 by Harris and his colleagues and also by research scientists in the Merck Laboratories, USA.

Sources

Biotin is widely distributed in animals and plants and good natural sources of it are yeast, liver, kidney, egg yolk, milk, peas, molasses and cereals. Small amounts of biotin occur in many vegetables and fruits.

Research workers have discovered that there is a basic protein in egg white which combines with biotin and prevents it being utilized by the body. This basic protein has been named 'avidin' because of the avidity with which it combines with biotin.

After avidin and biotin have formed a complex it cannot be broken down by the body's digestive processes; only by cooking or irradiation. For this reason eggs should never be eaten raw, but always cooked.

Losses occur during cooking processes, mainly due to a leaching out into the cooking water or other fluids. The drying of milk causes serious losses of the vitamin but now this is known, such milks are supplemented with biotin. A substantial part of the daily intake of biotin is supplied from synthesis in the intestine by the bacteria there. This is suggested by the finding that the quantity of the vitamin excreted is often higher than that eaten in the diet. Naturally this important source is reduced dramatically by antibiotic therapy which destroys the 'friendly' bacteria, so it is wise to supplement with the vitamin when being treated with these drugs.

Daily Requirements

Daily intakes of biotin have been put at between 150 and 300 micrograms, but absolute requirements are difficult to assess because the vitamin is supplied also by the normal intestinal bacteria.

Probable Functions in Man

Biotin is now known to be a coenzyme for a wide variety of body functions. It is required in the production of energy from carbohydrates, fats and proteins and in the conversion of these nutrients to important body substances. One specific function of biotin is in the metabolism of the essential polyunsaturated fatty acids (vitamin F) and when it is deficient, changes are reflected in the skin and hair because these tissues require vitamin F. For example, in babies, seborrheic dermatitis can be helped either by linoleic acid (vitamin F) or biotin. Hence the vitamin is needed for growth and the maintenance of healthy skin, hair, sweat glands, nerves, bone marrow and the glands producing sex hormones.

Deficiency Ailments

A deficiency of biotin in man causes muscular pain, poor appetite, dry skin, a disturbed nervous system, lack of energy and sleeplessness.

Laboratory animals deprived of biotin lost their

fur, especially around the eyes, suffered from an itchy dermatitis, retarded growth and a spastic gait. Such animals are susceptible to heart and lung ailments. Biotin appears to be essential for reproduction and lactation in mice. Puppies fed on a diet lacking in biotin, suffered from a progressive paralysis.

Biotin is considered by some research scientists to activate lysozyme, the bacteria-digesting antienzyme that is found in tears, mucus and body fluids.

Therapeutic Use

There have been trials of high potency biotin in skin complaints, alopecia and other scalp conditions and some success has been reported. Apart from these studies, however, there do not seem to be any specific complaints that will respond to biotin apart from those due to simple deficiency.

Toxicity of Biotin

Despite daily intakes of 10 milligrams per day by babies there were no toxic reactions reported. Levels above this have been tolerated by adults with no problems.

CHOLINE

Choline has been known to science since 1849. In 1939, Best and Riddell showed that the ailment known as fatty liver could be remedied by giving choline to sufferers. Liver normally contains only between 5 and 7 per cent of its weight in fat, but in the absence of choline this proportion can increase to as much as 50 per cent. These fatty deposits, when present in excess, adversely affect the functioning of this vital organ and the ill-effects are soon felt. Fatty liver can be a feature of many diseases, including diabetes, alcoholism and protein-deficiency.

Function of Choline

Choline is defined as a lipotropic factor, which means that it prevents fat accumulating in the vital organs of the body by facilitating the transport of these fats within the body. When fats are transported from these organs, they do so in the form of complex substances called phospholipids. These are composed of fats, phosphorus, sugar and choline in combination. Lack of choline prevents this efficient fat-mobilizing system from functioning so there is a build-up of unwanted fat in parts of the body where it should not be. This includes blood vessels as well as places like the heart, liver, kidney and brain. Supplementing with choline not only prevents this abnormal accumulation of fat but actually clears it. This role for choline has been proved in animals and confirmed in human beings in studies as long ago as 1951 (*Journal of the American Medical Association*).

Sources of Choline

Choline is present in many animal and plant tissues, good food sources being wheatgerm, liver, brains, kidney and eggs. The richest source of choline is, however, lecithin. Milk is a poor source of choline. The following vegetables contain choline: soya beans, asparagus, Brussels sprouts, cabbage, carrots, peas, spinach, turnips and potatoes.

The amino acid methionine can be converted by

the body into choline, hence the body is capable of making its own to a certain extent but this depends upon the availability of the precursors of choline, amongst which is methionine. Ample supplies of methionine are therefore necessary and these may be lacking when on a poor protein diet.

Choline and Healthy Nerves

Choline is essential in maintaining the myelin sheath of nerves which, as mentioned previously, acts like an insulator round an electric cable. In addition to this, however, choline is the precursor of a nerve substance called acetylcholine. This acetylcholine acts as a chemical messenger, relaying nerve impulses from one nerve to the next or from nerve to muscle. Lack of choline means that acetylcholine cannot be produced so nerve functions deteriorate, with serious consequences.

It is for this reason that choline has recently been tried as a treatment for senile dementia. One aspect of this complaint is an increasing inability of the individual to produce acetylcholine. By supplying massive doses of choline it appears that it is possible to overcome the metabolic block between choline and acetylcholine. Studies reported in *The Lancet* in 1978 claimed a dramatic improvement in patients suffering from senile dementia when they were given 25 grams of lecithin daily, providing 900 mg of choline. Lecithin is preferred to choline itself as it is better utilized by the body.

Choline and Diseases of Fat Metabolism

Choline's role as a pipotropic agent has led to its use in diseases where fat metabolism has gone wrong.

In 1950, Drs L. M. Morrison and W. F. Gonzalez of the Los Angeles County Hospital reported that patients suffering from coronary occlusion or coronary thrombosis have derived great benefit from being given choline. At the same time the amount of cholesterol in their blood decreased. Choline has also provided benefit in those suffering from angina, thrombosis or stroke when these diseases have developed through a defect in handling fat, leading to its deposition in blood vessel walls.

High blood pressure has also responded in some individuals treated with choline. According to a report in *Journal of Vitaminology* in 1957 typical symptoms of palpitation, dizziness and headaches disappeared within two weeks of treatment together with a reduction of blood pressure to normal.

Daily Requirements

According to Drs Bicknell and Prescott, very little choline is excreted by the body. The requirement of choline in the average human diet is high, namely approximately 650 mg daily. This is in addition to that produced by the body itself.

INOSITOL

Inositol was first discovered to be a food factor in 1850, but almost a century was to pass before it was recognized as a B complex vitamin.

Inositol appears to be associated with choline and biotin. In an experiment carried out by Dr Woolley of the Rockefeller Institute, USA, in 1940, mice were given a diet that lacked only inositol. They ceased to grow and hair fell out until parts of their bodies became almost denuded of fur. After pure inositol, or the inositol contained in yeast or liver was fed to the mice, new hair grew within eighteen days. Experiments with other animals gave similar results.

In a report in the *American Heart Journal* (1949) Drs Leinwand and Moore found that a daily intake of inositol of 3 grams resulted in a reduction of blood fats and cholesterol in patients suffering from atherosclerosis. Similar claims were made in the *Journal of the American Medical Association* (1953) by Drs Sherber and Levites but in their patients, both inositol and choline were given in quantities of 1 gram of each.

Function of Inositol

As with choline, inositol aids in the metabolism of fats and in its absence fatty liver develops in experimental animals. In some cases, inositol supplementation is able to remove excess fat from the livers of people suffering from fatty liver.

There is a high concentration of inositol in the lens of the eye and in the muscles of the heart, which seems to imply that inositol is important to clear the vision and to promote healthy heart action. It appears necessary too in maintaining a healthy gastro-intestinal tract since the cells here are very rich in inositol. Inositol has been used with benefit by those whose hair was falling out. It appears also to function in maintaining healthy skin and muscular tissue, since mild skin complaints and mild inflammation of the muscles have been induced by inositol deficiency and these complaints have cleared up by giving the compound.

Adelle Davis, American nutritional scientist,

writes in *Let's Eat Right to Keep Fit* that an inositol lack is linked with coronary heart ailments, also that an inositol deficiency causes constipation, eczema and abnormalities of the eyes.

Dr W. H. Eddy in *Vitaminology* says that caffeine creates an inositol shortage in the body. Caffeine is contained in coffee and tea, and in Australia the consumption of both is very high. Caffeine is also added to some popular American soft drinks.

The probable daily requirement of inositol in man is around 1000 mg.

Inositol and the Nervous System

The brain and spinal cord nerves contain very high concentrations of inositol and part of it is found, like choline, in the myelin sheath. Inositol, however, has some function apart from a structural one, according to Dr Pfieffer of the Brain Bio Centre, Princetown, New Jersey. He found different responses of inositol on the brain wave patterns between normal and schizophrenic people. Inositol appeared to have a similar anti-anxiety effect to that of mild tranquilizing drugs like Librium and could indeed replace these drugs in some people. It is therefore highly possible that anxiety, irritability and over-activity may be related to a simple deficiency of inositol or due to some blockage of inositol metabolism.

Sources

This vitamin is supplied in heart muscle, liver, yeast, wheatgerm, oatmeal and molasses, but it also occurs in beans, peas, grapefruit, oranges, peaches, peanuts, potatoes, spinach, strawberries, tomatoes, turnips and some other vegetables. Like choline, inositol is richly contained in lecithin.

Inositol is present in all animal and plant tissues. The highest concentration in animal tissues occurs in muscle, brain, red blood cells, heart and kidneys. In cereals, much of the inositol present occurs in phytic acid — a complex of inositol with phosphorus. Some of this is degraded to give free inositol but the amount is not known. In the body, under the influence of body cells and intestinal bacteria, glucose is converted to inositol but, again, the extent is unknown. Diet therefore still remains an important source of inositol.

4

Vitamin C (Ascorbic Acid)

The discovery of vitamin C was the result of scientific investigations made to find the cause and cure of scurvy, which plagued mankind for centuries.

In 1912 Funk postulated a scurvy-preventing vitamin, vitamin C, and efforts were made to isolate it from orange and lemon juice, which had proved most effective against scurvy.

Zilva, in 1924, obtained a 300-fold concentration and in 1928 Gyorgyi isolated vitamin C, which he called hexuronic acid, from cabbage and the adrenal cortex.

The structural formula of vitamin C was established in 1933 by Haworth and Hirst who synthesized it in the same year, when it was given the more fitting name of ascorbic acid. This is a condensation of anti-scorbutic acid, meaning preventing scurvy.

Function of Vitamin C
Research indicates that vitamin C is essential to form and maintain healthy connective tissue. The trillions of cells that make up the body are held together by this tissue, called collagen, and when it breaks down, not only the supporting connective tissue, but the cartilage, ligaments and walls of

blood vessels weaken. This facilitates the admission of invading bacteria and viruses that cause infections. Vitamin C assists the body to deal effectively with these foreign attackers, because strong connective tissue offers a powerful obstacle. Vitamin C also strengthens their natural enemies, the phagocytes and antibodies.

The antibodies produced by the liver which help to make bacteria harmless, need vitamin C to render them vigorous and active. Antibodies also detoxify allergens which enter the bloodstream in the form of pollens, dust, dandruff, and foreign proteins in foodstuffs, vaccines and serums, giving rise to such allergies as hay fever, hives, eczema, asthma, etc.

Recent research has implicated vitamin C in the metabolism of fats including cholesterol. Guinea-pigs, like man, require an external source of vitamin C so they are one of the few animal species that lend themselves to research into the vitamin. When deprived of vitamin C the cholesterol levels in the blood of guinea-pigs increase. Fat is deposited in the walls of blood vessels, particularly those of the heart and brain. In addition, these animals show a greater tendency to form gallstones. Observations indicate that in human beings too, low vitamin C levels in the body lead to increased cholesterol and deposition of fat. One way in which ascorbic acid functions in controlling fats is to stimulate the breakdown and hence excretion of cholesterol.

If we wish to sum up the function of vitamin C in the body in a few words it can be described as an anti-oxidant. This simply means that it prevents other compounds being oxidized, i.e. destroyed or made unavailable. A prime example is iron, which exists in two forms called ferrous and fernic. The iron in food and in the intestine must be in the ferrous form to be assimilated and vitamin C ensures that the iron remains thus. Hence the vitamin contributes to the prevention of iron-deficiency anaemia. At the same time ascorbic acid is essential to convert folic acid into its active form, folinic acid. If this does not happen, the result is another type of anaemia due to lack of active folic acid. Perhaps it is not surprising then that anaemia is one of the commonest symptoms of vitamin C deficiency.

Vitamin C is also concerned with the conversion of amino acids to substances in the brain needed for normal brain and nervous functions. Lack of the vitamin causes mental symptoms, particularly in the aged, and treatment with ascorbic acid often restores mental alertness in these people. The stress hormones of the body require vitamin C for their production within the glands. In both of these functions vitamin C is acting as a reducing agent or anti-oxidant.

For Bones and Teeth

Vitamin C promotes healthy bone growth and the knitting of bone fractures. When this vitamin is lacking, bones become soft, porous or brittle and break readily after a minor fall or injury. Bone fractures heal badly when there is a deficiency of vitamin C.

Degenerative changes occur in the teeth and gums when the diet lacks this vitamin. The bone of the teeth becomes injured and the enamel is weakened. The gums become inflamed and recede from the teeth, making the latter appear unusually long. The teeth, having no firm support, loosen in their sockets and pyorrhea pockets develop at the base of the teeth, forming areas of infection.

The rate of efficiency of wound healing depends upon the amount of vitamin C and protein that is concentrated in the tissues. In diseases such as TB collagen be produced, to prevent further breakdown of tissue with likely re-infection. Hence the rate at which any healing process takes place depends upon the ability of the body tissue affected to produce new collagen. Collagen, like all proteins, is a complex structure made up of amino acids, some 22 in all, but it is unique in containing a high proportion of two of them called proline and hydroxyproline. Hydroxyproline is not supplied in the diet and the only way the body can get it is from proline. This conversation is completely under the control of vitamin C. In the absence of the vitamin, therefore, hydroxyproline is not produced and the resulting collagen is weak. The healing process is thus slow and inefficient. Bone has a high content of collagen so its rate of mending after fracture is also dependent on vitamin C being present in adequate concentration.

For Muscles

Ever since the symptoms of scurvy were first described in the mid-seventeenth century, the consistent common factor in the early signs of the disease is the appearance of muscle fatigue. The reason is that the contraction of the muscle requires the presence of the muscle component carnitine. Carnitine itself is produced within the body from an amino acid we eat called lysine. This conversion of lysine to carnitine is completely dependent upon vitamin C. Lack of the vitamin means lack of carnitine and the end result is inefficient contraction of the muscle, leading to fatigue and tiredness. It is because this vitamin is so important for muscle contraction that it is a popular supplement for athletes.

The Capillaries

The capillaries, hair-like blood vessels that ramify into almost every part of the body, become fragile and break down when vitamin C is lacking. When this happens, blood escapes into the tissues, bone marrow joints, etc., leading to rheumatic and other ailments.

The function of the capillaries is to carry nutrients and oxygen to the cells and to carry away waste products therefrom. When supplies of nutrients and oxygen fail to reach cells, due to broken capillaries, those cells die in a matter of seconds. Dead cells have no protection against bacteria. Instead, such cells actually foster the growth of harmful invaders of the bloodstream and enable bacteria to gain access to other parts of the body. Bacteria may thus reach the joints to cause arthritis; the kidneys to result in kidney ailments, or the heart to give rise to rheumatic heart disease.

People who bruise easily, or are subject to nose bleeding are almost certain to be suffering from fragile capillaries, which require vitamin C to nourish and strengthen them. This effect of the vitamin upon capillaries can be observed in the tiny blood vessels of the tongue. When these change in appearance it may be a sign of an impending heart attack or stroke, according to Dr Geoffrey Taylor, formerly Professor of Medicine at the University of Lahore. Such changes also appear in scurvy and are some of the earliest signs of vitamin C deficiency. It is not without significance that deaths from heart attacks and stroke increase during winter months when vitamin C intake is usually at its lowest level.

It is likely that vitamin C does not function alone in maintaining the integrity of the minor blood vessels. The bioflavanoids appear to complement this action of the vitamin. In nature, bioflavanoids always accompany ascorbic acid, so as long as we look to natural fruit and vegetable sources for our vitamin C we are receiving bioflavanoids as well, and in the right proportion.

Vitamin C Losses and Increased Requirements

Several drugs cause vitamin C to be lost rapidly by excretion, namely, aspirin, the barbiturates, salicylates, sulphanilamide, insulin, thyroid extract, atrophin, antihistamine drugs, adrenaline, and the contraceptive pill. However, of all these drugs the two most commonly used, and for prolonged periods, are aspirin and the components of the contraceptive pill.

The increased losses of the vitamin induced by aspirin can only be compensated for by taking between 200 and 300 mg of the vitamin for each aspirin tablet swallowed. Beneficial effects of vitamin C when taken with aspirin include better absorption and thus faster action of the drug and a reduced tendency to gastric bleeding that is a feature of aspirin taking in some people. The contraceptive pill does not cause increased excretion of vitamin C but appears to increase requirements. A daily intake of 500 mg of the vitamin is sufficient to overcome the low blood levels induced by the contraceptive pill.

The habits of smoking tobacco and drinking alcohol both increase the requirements of vitamin C. The poison present in tobacco smoke, called acetaldehyde, is also produced within the body from alcohol, and its effect is not only to cause increased excretion of the vitamin but also to destroy it. It has been suggested by Dr W. J. MacCormack, writing in *Archives of Paediatrics* that each cigarette destroys 25 mg of vitamin C so every smoker can take sufficient supplementary vitamin to overcome any possible deficiency. Alcohol drinkers need at least 1000 mg of supplementary vitamin C daily to overcome the ravages induced by their drinking habits, according to Dr Spince at the Veterans' Hospital, Pennsylvania, USA.

Any condition that gives rise to stress also requires an increased intake of vitamin C to maintain normal blood levels. The reason probably lies in the role of the vitamin in the production of the anti-stress hormones by the adrenal glands. Stress situations deplete the glands of their hormones and their level cannot be maintained without adequate vitamin C. Two, three or even five times the usual daily intake of the vitamin may thus be required when under stress, so 500 mg per day is not unusual.

Sources of Vitamin C

Vitamin C is widely distributed throughout nature,

but the richest sources are fruit and vegetables. Pride of place amongst readily available foods must go to blackcurrants, broccoli spears, kale, parsley and red and green peppers. Even richer, however, are the more exotic fruits like acerola cherry and camu-camu plum. Excellent sources amongst the more common vegetables are Brussels sprouts, cabbage, cauliflower, chives and mustard greens. Citrus fruits are good providers of the vitamin, one large orange containing 50 mg. In this country potatoes, although not particularly rich in the vitamin, represent an important source of vitamin C mainly because of the large amounts eaten in the daily diet.

Losses during Cooking

Vitamin C is the most sensitive of the vitamins and it is easily destroyed by storage of food, food refining, food processing and cooking on both the commercial and domestic levels. Losses on simple storage are due to enzymic oxidation of the vitamin and are accelerated by bruising and handling of the fruit and vegetables. Alkalis like baking powder are particularly detrimental to vitamin C. The water-soluble nature of ascorbic acid means that it leaches away during cooking processes but these losses are recoverable if cooking fluids are utilized.

Therapeutic Uses of Vitamin C

Vitamin C can be used with benefit for colds, hay fever, influenza, catarrh, asthma, bronchitis, sinusitis and other infections of the respiratory system. Clinical trials have indicated that intakes to prevent respiratory infections are in the region of 500 to

1000 mg of the vitamin daily. If there is an infection present, daily intakes must be increased to 3 to 5 grams while the infection persists, but may be gradually reduced afterwards to the base level of 500 to 1000 mg.

There have also been claims that high potency vitamin C can complement other treatments of cancer. Intakes of 10 grams or more daily are required. Vitamin C is believed to function in one way by strengthening the collagen around the tumour and thus preventing its spread. The vitamin can also neutralize the substances present in the food we eat that are capable of causing cancer. Similarly when these carcinogens are produced within body cells, vitamin C can exert a protective action by destroying them.

We have seen that adequate vitamin C must be present for effective healing of wounds either accidental or surgery-produced. The vitamin is also useful to reduce bruising and may be helpful to decrease the swelling of varicose veins.

Daily Requirements

These vary tremendously depending upon which authority recommends them. The UK and Australia recommended allowances are 30 mg, but those of the USA are 60 mg. It is quite likely that both these figures are low under present-day conditions and between 100 and 150 mg at least should be aimed at daily. Babies should receive at least 50 mg in their diets.

Toxicity

Despite the occasional report to the contrary,

vitamin C is generally accepted as non-toxic. Up to 10 grams daily have been taken for long periods without any side-effects and intakes of 30 to 40 grams for a short time have been taken quite safely.

5

Vitamin D

Cod liver oil was in use a century ago as a remedy for rickets — a disease of children and marked by faulty bone formation. In adults, this condition is called osteomalacia.

In 1918, Mellanby produced rickets in dogs by giving them an unbalanced diet and he remedied the disease with cod liver oil. At the time, it was thought that vitamin A was the curative factor in rickets. Research by McCollum in 1922 demonstrated that vitamin A given in foods other than cod liver oil, failed to cure rickets. McCollum then destroyed the vitamin A in cod liver oil by bubbling hot air through it and found that oil so treated still cured rickets, although it had no value for eye infections which normally respond to vitamin A.

In 1919, research proved that the action of ultraviolet rays in sunshine, or the light from a mercury-vapour quartz lamp were also curative in rickets.

Vitamin D was synthesized in crystalline form in 1935, and since then about twenty different forms of this vitamin have been investigated, but only two are in practical use, namely, vitamins D_2 and D_3.

Sources

Only a very few foods provide vitamin D. The best sources are the liver oils of fish which obtain the vitamin by ingesting plankton living near the surface of the sea. These tiny organisms are exposed to the sunlight which provides them with vitamin D. Once the fish have eaten the plankton, they absorb the vitamin and store it in the liver. Other sources of vitamin D are dairy products, with eggs and butter representing the highest concentration. The only meat with worthwhile quantities of vitamin D present is liver. Human breast milk provides enough vitamin D to prevent deficiency in the baby, but cow's milk contains much less. For this reason, in the USA and Canada all cows' milk is fortified with the vitamin, but this practice is not usual in Europe, where only margarine is fortified with vitamin D.

All vitamin D is produced by the action of ultraviolet light on waxy precursors called provitamin D. There are two types. In the oil glands of the skin there is a compound called 7-dehydrocholesterol, itself produced by the body from cholesterol. When ultraviolet light from the sun or from some other source like a sunlamp falls upon 7-dehydrocholesterol, vitamin D_3 is produced. This eventually finds its way to the bloodstream and thence is distributed throughout the body where it exerts its functions.

When dogs and cats lick their coats, it is considered that they thereby absorb vitamin D, as do birds when they preen their feathers. Test rats which have developed rickets from lack of vitamin D in their diet, are cured if they are allowed to lick their coats, when exposed to sunlight. Animals which hibernate, such as the hedgehog, do not do so when given vitamin D. Under natural conditions with the approach of winter and waning sunlight the animal's supply of vitamin D declines. This causes it to 'burn' less blood sugar and become torpid. Its metabolism slows down and its food consumption is very low, whereas hedgehogs given vitamin D, developed too much energy to permit hibernation.

Steenbock showed in 1924 that vitamin D_3 can be added to foods such as milk and margarine by exposing them to ultraviolet rays. They thus become irradiated. Vitamin D_3 is also known as cholecalciferol, i.e. produced from cholesterol.

Clouds, fog, haze and smog prevent the sun's ultraviolet rays from reaching the earth and surveys made in cities where bad weather conditions often prevail, reveal more cases of rickets than cities which have clearer skies and more hours of sunlight annually.

The other widely-used form of vitamin D is called vitamin D_2 or ergocalciferol. This is manufactured by exposing ergosterol, a cholesterol-like substance found in yeast, to ultraviolet light. Irradiation of ergosterol gives rise to several substances, some of which are toxic, so that the conditions of exposure to the ultraviolet light are critical and must be carefully controlled. Vitamin D_2 is widely used in supplements, particulary by vegetarians and vegans because it has not been produced from an animal source. It is just as active as naturally-produced vitamin D_3 that is synthesized in the skin.

The vitamin D we require to ensure health is thus supplied from two sources, the diet and ultraviolet light. If we allow plenty of sunlight to fall on large areas of skin, enough vitamin D is manufactured and dietary sources become less important. During winter months when the light is less intense and the skin is covered for warmth we rely upon dietary vitamin D for our needs. However, it has been calculated by Dr Looms that the pink cheeks of a European infant (area about 20 sq. cms) can synthesize daily 10 micrograms of vitamin D_3 — the daily requirements — if exposure to light is adequate.

Vitamin D and the Teeth

Mrs May Mellanby, wife of the scientist who produced experimental rickets in dogs, carried out extensive research to establish the relationship between vitamin D and the teeth. She found that even mild forms of rickets interfere with the normal development of infants' teeth, also the structure and shape of the jawbone, causing narrow dental arches, crooked, overlapping and protruding teeth, defective bite, faulty alignment of teeth, etc.

According to Davis, vitamin D helps to prevent tooth decay and plays an important part in preventing pyorrhea.

Functions of Vitamin D

Vitamin D is considered to control an enzyme called phosphatase, which appears essential to bone formation. The function of this enzyme is to act upon fats and sugars that are combined with phosphorus and to release the phosphorus for bone-building purposes. This detached phosphorus then forms a union with calcium brought along by the bloodstream and both minerals share in building and hardening the bone structure, which in young children is a pliable, gristly substance called collagen.

The foregoing complicated processes fail to occur when vitamin D is lacking in the diet. Instead, the enzyme, phosphatase, leaves the bone foundation and enters the bloodstream. Phosphorus is then not released from fats and sugars and is unavailable to combine with calcium, hence these minerals are not deposited in the young bones and growth may cease. Half the phosphorus in the body is normally found in the bones.

Should inadequate vitamin D be supplied, some phosphatase is present, but bone growth is slowed down and the formation of teeth is delayed and disorganized.

The vitamin D formed in the skin or supplied in the diet is not the active form of the vitamin. Once it reaches the liver it is converted to another form known as 25-hydroxy vitamin D (abbreviated to 25-OH-D). This is the form in which it is transported in the bloodstream but it is still not active. The active form is called 1,25-dihydroxy vitamin D (abbreviated to $1,25\text{-}(OH)_2\text{-}D$) and this is produced only in the kidneys. It is $1,25\text{-}(OH)_2\text{-}D$ that regulates calcium and phosphorus metabolism.

There are certain diseases where vitamin D is not absorbed from the diet, as where the conversion to 25-OH-D and $1,25\text{-}(OH)_2\text{-}D$ does not happen and the end result is all the symptoms of vitamin D deficiency. If the conversion does not happen it is futile treating with vitamin D and the only therapy is to supply $1,25\text{-}(OH)_2\text{-}D$, and this by injection. The discovery and the use of this active form of vitamin D has revolutionized the treatment of some diseases produced by deficiency of the vitamin which were hitherto refractory.

Deficiency Ailments

In some respects, vitamin D is the most important of all the vitamins, for deformity of the bone framework in childhood, due to a shortage of this vitamin can cause irreparable injury which continues throughout life, because once the bones harden the 'die is cast' for good or ill.

Children deprived of calcium and phosphorus in their diet also become stunted and develop bone malformations. Following World War II and the period of malnutrition which ensued, many children in Germany and Austria showed symptoms such as curvature of the spine, bow legs, knock knees, etc. Even children in their late teens were affected. The disease is known as rickets in children and it is usually the result of a combination of poor diet and lack of sunshine. Once this was realized, in the 1930s, the disease practically disappeared in the UK. Sadly, the disease has now reappeared and is almost exclusively confined to the coloured immigrant population. No one is quite sure of the reasons for this but they are probably social, environmental and dietary. The simplest prevention is a daily supplement for these people.

In adults, the equivalent vitamin D deficiency disease is called osteomalacia. The bones do not buckle as they do in rickets because they are already fully formed but they still lack calcium and phosphorus and become very brittle.

The metabolic functions of vitamin D (in the form of 1,25-$(OH)_2$-D on calcium and phosphorus metabolism are now well established. They are:

1   it promotes calcium absorption from the diet in the upper part of the small intestine;
2   it acts on bone to mobilize calcium from the bone reservoir and also allows bone to take up the mineral;
3   it facilitates phosphorus absorption (in the form of phosylate) in similar fashions to those of calcium.

Vitamin D and Energy

One of the functions of vitamin D is to release energy within the body. Phosphorus carries blood sugar through the intestinal wall, as well as to the liver, which stores it as glycogen. Blood sugar is 'burned' to supply energy and when vitamin D is lacking, sugar cannot combine with phosphorus, hence energy flags.

Research has shown that children who lack vitamin D burn less blood sugar and display less energy than normal children. The combination of sugar and phosphorus in the muscles is reduced, children in the former case lose blood sugar in the urine, and their blood contains more than normal amounts of sugar. There is thus an incomplete storage of blood sugar as glycogen, and an incomplete absorption of it in providing energy.

Davis raises the question whether some of those who crave sweets are not actually lacking vitamin

D, because when the body cannot use sugar, it expresses this deficiency in a craving for sweets. It is possible too that some people who lack vitamin D during winter months, owing to inadequate exposure to sunshine or infrequent sunny days, may become short of energy for this reason.

Vitamin D is important to maintain healthy eyes. Experiments with puppies have shown that when fed on a diet deficient in vitamin D, changes occur in the eyes, comparable with changes noticed in the eyes of adults and children. These alterations give rise to shortsightedness or myopia, an inability to bend light rays sufficiently.

Effect of Sun's Rays

During the winter months, owing to the sun's lower altitude, fewer ultraviolet rays reach the earth. Experiments with rats kept on diets to induce rickets, have shown that only five minutes of mid-summer sun is required to keep them free from rickets, whereas almost three hours of mid-winter sun are needed.

McCollum states: 'Even in clear weather, and in the country, sunlight contains no appreciable ultraviolet light, except when the sun is above thirty degrees from the horizon.'

Ordinary window glass and dark, heavy clothing exclude ultraviolet rays. Dark-complexioned people do not absorb as much vitamin D as those with lighter coloured skins, and people with heavy suntan, cannot absorb vitamin D. Negro children are susceptible to rickets on account of their colour.

The too frequent scrubbing of horses with soap and water can produce rickets. This is due to the removal from their skin of the provitamin irradiated 7-dehydrocholesterol. Soap has a more severe effect upon 7-dehydrocholesterol than water alone.

Taking Vitamin D

The use of paraffin oil as a laxative prevents the fat-soluble vitamins, namely, A, E, F and K. Moreover, it damages the liver, according to Drs Bicknell and Prescott. These authorities also state that fluoride (used in some public water supplies to prevent dental decay in children) retards the action of vitamin D in warding off rickets.

The best source of vitamin D other than sunlight is, as we have stated, fish liver oil. This can be obtained in capsule form (together with vitamin A) by those who dislike taking fish liver oil as such.

Like other fat-soluble vitamins, vitamins D and A are best assimilated after a meal containing some fatty food, such as butter, cheese, milk, etc.

Recommended Intakes

One characteristic of vitamin D is the narrow gap between the nutrient requirements and the toxic dose. The usual daily needs are 10 micrograms but as little as five times this have led to toxic symptoms in infants and adults. Typical symptoms are loss of appetite followed by nausea and vomiting. Thirst and frequent passing of water soon follow. Constipation and then diarrhoea become a feature of upset in the gastro-intestinal tract. Head pains and joint pains then appear. The child becomes thin, irritable and depressed eventually progressing into a coma which may end in death. The usual daily requirement of 10 micrograms is also expressed as 40 IU.

6

Vitamin E (Alpha Tocopherol)

Vitamin E was first isolated from wheatgerm oil by Evans and others in 1936. Its existence was foreshadowed as a dietary factor by Mattil and Conklin in 1920, and in 1922 Evans and Bishop proved that it is essential for normal reproduction.

In 1931, Goettsche and Pappenheimer demonstrated that laboratory guinea pigs and rabbits developed muscular dystrophy when deprived of vitamin E and in 1938 Bicknell started to treat children affected by this ailment with vitamin E. Other workers followed his example, with some limited success.

Vitamin E occurs as alpha, beta, gamma and delta tocopherols but if we regard the activity of the alpha as 100 per cent, that of the others is 40 per cent, 8 per cent and 1 per cent respectively in biological tests. However, as an anti-oxidant (i.e. in its ability to prevent rancidity of fats) delta tocopherol is the most active. Most of the studies of vitamin E in animals and people have been carried out on alpha tocopherol, so in most respects the vitamin is equated for alpha tocopherol.

Alpha tocopherol exists in two forms known as dextro (or d-alpha) tocopherol and laevo (or l-alpha) tocopherol. The naturally-occurring form is d-alpha tocopherol; the synthetic is referred to as dl-alpha tocopherol which means it is an equal mixture of both d- and l- forms. Only the d-alpha form is biologically active, so is more potent than the synthetic one which contains only 50 per cent of this form.

In tablets and capsules vitamin E is usually present as alpha tocopheryl acetate and alpha tocopheryl succinate. These are known as esters and they are used because in these forms vitamin E is more stable. Similar considerations of potency apply, however, and in all cases the natural d-alpha form of the vitamin is more active in the body than the dl-alpha synthetic type.

Vitamin E is rapidly and completely destroyed by rancid fats and inorganic iron preparations but only when these are of the ferric type. Ferrous iron does not affect vitamin E and fortunately most of the supplements that combine the vitamin with iron present the mineral in the ferrous form. Hence they are perfectly stable and safe. One of the functions of vitamin E is the protect vitamin A, also the B complex vitamins and biotin against destruction by rancid fats. People with over-active thyroid glands need more than normal daily requirements of vitamin E. There is evidence that it is intimately concerned with the central nervous system.

Sources

The richest natural sources of vitamin E are the vegetable oils, with concentrations per 100 grams varying from wheatgerm (190 mg) to peanut (22 mg). The exceptions are coconut oil, linseed oil and olive oil which have very little. Unrefined cereals provide useful amounts of the vitamin in the diet with oatmeal and muesli containing between 3 and 4 mg per 100 grams. There is a small amount of vitamin E in lettuce, tomatoes, carrots, egg yolk, fish roe and nuts. Vitamin E is fat-soluble and is not harmed by cooking. All fruits and most meats contain less than one milligram of vitamin E per 100 grams. Some vegetables like sweet potato, turnip greens, peas and beans provide between 1 and 4 mg per 100 gram in the raw state but this is reduced to less than a milligram after cooking, blanching and frying. Converting wholegrain wheat into white flour causes the loss of almost 90 per cent of the vitamin E content. Unfortunately when edible vegetable oils are hydrogenated (hardened), as is the current practice in producing hard margarines, most of the vitamin E is destroyed by the process. The vitamin is absent from animal fats like lard and dripping. Solvent-extracted vegetable oils contain less vitamin E than the cold-pressed variety because the tocopherol tends to be left behind after solvent extraction and it is easily destroyed when the solvent is removed. Butter and cream contain almost no vitamin E. Dried and pasteurized milk may contain no vitamin E, according to Bicknell and Prescott, so that artificially fed babies will receive inadequate supplies of the vitamin.

During the steel-roller milling of flour, the vitamin E content is removed, which doubtless explains the tremendous increase in degenerative diseases since this method of milling was adopted, about a century ago.

Functions

According to Mattill, more vitamin E occurs in the body than any other vitamin. Vitamin E appears essential for muscular health (and the heart is a muscle); it helps to utilize fat; it is concentrated in the pituitary, adrenals and sex glands; it prevents vitamin A, linoleic acid and possibly other nutrients from destruction by oxygen within the body, and it performs several other important functions. Mattill says of vitamin E: 'Perhaps no other of the vitamins mysteriously affects so many and so varied bodily processes.'

The main function of vitamin E is best summed up by describing it as an anti-oxidant and as a main protective vitamin in the body. As we have seen, the other main protecting agent is vitamin C but this is water-soluble. Hence vitamin E tends to protect the fatty areas of the body because it dissolves in fat. Vitamin C acts in the aqueous media of the body. Modern research results suggest that both vitamins C and E are also mutually protective.

The Role of Selenium

Recent studies have indicated that the trace mineral selenium acts in conjunction with vitamin E in its anti-oxidant functions. Both occur as coenzymes in certain enzyme systems. Weight for weight, selenium is far more active as an anti-oxidant than vitamin E but as the two complement each other both must be present in adequate quantities for optimum health.

Vitamin E Deficiency in Modern Diet

Davis points out that before wheat was milled by

the steel-roller process, the intake of vitamin E was estimated at 100 to 150 mg per head daily. Today, our foods supply only a tenth of this amount, or less.

Bicknell and Prescott say that there is only 4 to 8 mg of vitamin E in English food, and about 14 mg in the USA dietary. It is likely that Australian food is just as poor in vitamin E as American food.

Requirement

According to Horwitt, the minimum daily requirement of vitamin E is 30 mg. He has shown that anything less tends to result in haemolysis (destruction of red blood cells and loss of haemoglobin). Other research workers, namely, Engel, Harris, and Quaife, announced some years ago that the minimum daily human requirement of vitamin E is 30 mg. Vitamin E is virtually non-toxic and can be stored very efficiently by the body.

Many studies have now indicated that a woman's requirement of vitamin E can increase ten-fold during the menopause (i.e. up to 400 IU daily). As an individual gets older, vitamin E needs also increase and a daily intake of 300 to 400 IU is a wise investment for anyone.

Use for Heart Disease

The use of vitamin E for heart disease began in 1947 when Dr Evan Shute, of London, Ontario, Canada, treated his mother, then 71 years old, who was suffering from angina pectoris and water retention in the arms and legs (known as oedema). After five days of using vitamin E, the anginal pains vanished and the dropsical swellings, too. Dr Evan Shute and his brother, Dr Wilfred Shute, then began to use the vitamin E for other heart sufferers and have now treated over 40,000 patients, 80 per cent of whom obtained amazing benefit, most of them losing all the usual heart symptoms.

Many thousands of medical men all over the world are now prescribing vitamin E in the treatment of heart disease and high blood pressure, also for thrombosis, liver and kidney ailments, chronic leg ulcers, varicose veins, menopausal ills, serious burns, Buerger's disease, Reynaud's disease, and even early gangrene.

There is probably no vitamin that has lifted the shadow of despair from so many sufferers, as vitamin E.

Properties of Vitamin E
The following properties of vitamin E have been discovered:

1   It is a vasodilator, i.e. it dilates the capillaries and enables blood to flow freely into damaged, anaemic muscle tissue, thereby strengthening both the tissue and the nerves supplying it.
2   It decreases the oxygen requirements of muscle tissue by approximately 50 per cent. This is equivalent to an enhanced blood supply and diminishes pain and breathlessness.
3   It is an antithrombin, namely, it dissolves blood clots and prevents their formation, but does not interfere with the normal clotting of blood.
4   It prevents the formation of excessive scar tissue, and in some instances even melts

unwanted scar tissue.

5   It promotes urine excretion, hence it is useful in reducing oedema in heart patients.

6   It preserves the integrity of the walls of the capillaries, of vital importance to the damaged heart.

7   It increases collateral circulation, i.e. it promotes 'detour' blood channels around veins and arteries that are blocked.

8   It lends power and efficiency to muscle tissue, and has a most beneficial action upon tired, flagging heart muscle.

9   It improves the action of insulin in diabetes. There are many research papers confirming the value of alpha tocopherol in the treatment of diabetes for those receiving insulin or the oral drugs. However, diabetics usually develop blood circulation problems in later life but by taking vitamin E regularly whilst on treatment it is now suggested that these problems are reduced or averted.

10   It helps in regenerating new skin. A combination of oral vitamin E and direct application of a vitamin E cream or ointment to a scar or stretch marks will often help remove these unsightly blemishes. There are also reports that a similar combination approach will help heal leg ulcers and bed-sores.

Therapeutic Uses of Vitamin E

As well as the uses mentioned above, vitamin E has proved successful in other clinical conditions. At daily intakes of between 400 and 1000 IU the vitamin has been claimed to cure non-malignant breast cysts. One of its more widely quoted uses is in treating the condition known as intermittent claudication. This is due to a narrowing of the leg blood vessels resulting in sharp pains appearing after exercise. Vitamin E causes the blood vessels to dilate so allowing a free flow of blood to the limbs. By the same reasoning, the vitamin often helps relieve leg cramps, especially those occurring at night.

Toxicity

Vitamin E is virtually non-toxic but high doses (i.e. above 400 IU daily) should not be taken by those suffering from *uncontrolled* high blood–pressure.

7

Vitamin F
(Unsaturated Fatty Acids)

The essential unsaturated fatty acids, sometimes referred to as vitamin F, were first described by Burr and Burr in 1929, when they observed 'fat deficiency' disease in laboratory rats that had been deprived of certain fatty acids.

The disease manifested in a failure to put on weight. There was also a dryness and scurfiness which spread from the paws over the rest of their bodies. Cold weather accentuated this scurfiness — the kind that chaps hands. The rats also developed kidney stones and there were difficulties in reproduction. It was observed, too, that some relationship existed between the lack of unsaturated fatty acids and three members of the B complex vitamins, namely, pyridoxine, pantothenic acid and biotin.

Sources

The three polyunsaturated fatty acids are known as linoleic acid, linolenic acid, and arachidonic acid. These acids quickly become rancid when exposed to the air. They are found chiefly in cereal and vegetable fats and oils, namely, wheatgerm oil, safflower seed oil, cotton seed oil, rye-germ oil, maize-germ oil, sunflower seed oil, soya bean oil,

~anut oil, linseed oil, palm oil, olive oil, etc. but are poorly represented in such animal fats as butter, margarine, beef and mutton fat, lard, fish oil or milk.

Within the last few years the presence of other important essential polyunsaturated fatty acids have been demonstrated in foods. These are gamma linolenic acid (GLA) that is found only in oil of Evening Primrose, and eicosapentaenoic acid (EPA) that is confined to fish body oils. Both of these are metabolic products of linoleic, linolenic acid and arachidonic acids and are usually formed within the body. Lack of them can give rise to serious consequences resulting in specific illnesses so that their presence in the diet or as supplements then becomes of prime importance. According to the Lee Foundation for Nutritional Research, USA, unsaturated fatty acids reduce the incidence and duration of the common cold.

Deficiency Ailments

A number of human disorders seem to be associated with a deficiency of these fatty acids, namely, infantile eczema, adult eczema, dandruff, boils, acne, varicose ulcers, diarrhoeal conditions and underweight. They are also indicated when there is a dry skin, dry, brittle hair and nails, falling hair and kidney disease.

When the body is unable to synthesize sufficient gama linolenic acid some of the manifestations appear to be multiple sclerosis, atopic eczema and premenstrual problems. All of these complaints respond in some cases to oil of Evening Primrose, usually at an intake of 3000 mg daily. This supplies about 400 mg of GLA which is the active principle in the oil.

Lack of EPA is likely to increase the chances of blood clotting in blood vessels, giving rise to heart attacks and strokes. A diet that includes fatty fish will usually supply enough EPA, however, but this essential fatty acid is now available in capsule form.

Functions

It is also stated that the fatty acids function in the body by co-operating with vitamin D in making calcium available to the tissues; by aiding in the assimilation of phosphorus, and by nourishing the skin. The fatty acids seem to be related to the normal functioning of the adrenal glands, the reproductive process, and the thyroid gland. The essential polyunsaturated fatty acids are now known to be precursors of important hormones known as prostaglandins which in turn control many body processes. It is likely that the functions mentioned above are manifested through interaction between the glands and the various prostaglandins.

However, in addition to these metabolic functions the essential fatty acids also have an important structural role. They are an integral part of the myelin sheath, the fatty insulating layer around nerves. One of the features of multiple sclerosis is an incomplete myelin sheath and this is believed to cause some of the problems associated with the disease.

Cholesterol

Yet another task of the unsaturated fatty acids is to lower the cholesterol levels in the bloodstream. It is known that excessive cholesterol (derived from animal fats) tends to form deposits on the inner walls of blood vessels, thus restricting the lumen (opening) for blood to pass through. After a time, these deposits become silted over with minerals in the bloodstream and the blood vessels harden and lose their resilience. This condition gives rise to hardening of the arteries and high blood pressure. Should a hardened particle of cholesterol break away, it may plug an important artery, causing coronary occlusion or coronary thrombosis.

Lecithin
The polyunsaturated fatty acids are an integral part of a substance called lecithin, also found in egg yolk, liver and brains, which appears to be a homogenizing agent, i.e. it is able to break up fats and cholesterol into tiny droplets. In short, lecithin emulsifies cholesterol, and thereby prevents it from silting up blood vessels, or forming a thrombus.

Modern Foods Lack Lecithin
You may ask why are not the unsaturated fatty acids readily available in the ordinary diet? The answer is that modern foods are processed. Many edible vegetable fats are hydrogenated to change them from oily substances to hard fats that can be cut with a knife. This facilitates handling, packing and selling, but also destroys the essential fatty acids. Vegetable shortenings, processed cheeses, some peanut butters, cooking fats and margarines receive this hydrogenation treatment.

The human body can convert sugars to fats, but it cannot manufacture unsaturated fatty acids and must therefore obtain them from the foods we eat. These fatty acids contain what might be termed chemical 'hooks' which allow other substances to be linked to them. Thus, if oxygen becomes 'hooked', the fatty acids turn rancid. Cake mixes, pastry mixes, potato chips, popcorn and salted nuts, held too long in storage, are often rancid when purchased.

We have already seen what happens when hydrogen is 'hooked', namely, the fatty acids harden and also lose their lecithin content. The purpose of the 'hooks' is to permit essential fatty acids to combine with other nutrients, hence they are called 'unsaturated'.

Infantile Eczema

It is suspected that many cases of infantile eczema which occur soon after birth, are due to mothers avoiding vegetable and cereal oil fats, thus depriving their systems of lecithin needed to protect the baby against eczema. Adults with eczema, according to Davis, have been found to have abnormally small amounts of essential fatty acids in their blood.

Davis states that even psoriasis, one of the most stubborn eczema-like skin ailments, responds to lecithin. This authority also points out that overweight people, whose ankles, legs and thighs are swollen with oedema, can lose unnecessary pounds after taking lecithin. It is claimed that in many instances the overweight condition is solely due to the body being waterlogged.

The Need for Fat

Bloor considers that as many obese people refuse to

eat fats, the body changes sugars to fats more rapidly than normally in an effort to produce the missing nutrients. Fat people put on weight as a result and because they are usually excessively hungry they tend to overeat. It is known that fats are far more sustaining than sugary or starchy foods. Hence, by going short of fats there follows an over-indulgence in sugars and starches, both notorious weight producers for the obese.

Fat is needed to ensure the efficient production of bile and of the fat-splitting enzyme, lipase. When fat enters the intestine, the gall bladder empties itself through a duct that leads to the intestine. Should there be inadequate fat, too little bile is formed and the faulty emptying of the gall bladder may induce the production of gallstones. Moreover, the fat-soluble vitamins, A, D, E, F and K cannot be assimilated in the absence of fat and bile, and are lost to the body.

Fat is essential to health and a small amount of stored fat is needed for several purposes. Fat under the skin protects nerves and muscles and maintains warmth in cold weather. Fat around the kidneys supports them. A fat reserve is beneficial as a source of energy during sickness. It is only when fat is too abundant that it is objectionable. It is not so much the fat you eat, but the *kind of fat* that is important.

Value of Lecithin

Lecithin, contained in safflower seed oil, soya bean oil, sunflower seed oil, etc., besides helping to keep the skin and nails in health is a rich source of two B complex vitamins, choline and inositol. It also contains vitamins E and K, and zinc. Lecithin supplies an anti-oxidant that prevents rancidity, thereby preserving from destruction the fat-soluble vitamins already referred to, together with some of the B complex vitamins in our food and in the intestinal tract.

Because it helps to form the fatty myelin sheath around the nerves which both insulates and nourishes them, lecithin is used in the treatment of nerve troubles, nervous exhaustion, and brain fag.

Lecithin is also important to the health of the intestinal flora; it aids in keeping the body free from diarrhoea and other bowel ailments.

Some people find that any kind of oil taken from a spoon is nauseating, but lecithin is available in capsule form and in lecithin granules, to make good deficiencies.

8

Vitamin K

In 1931, a research scientist named McFarlane observed that fish-meal cured a haemorrhagic disease in chickens that had been fed upon diets deficient in fats. It was noticed, however, that when the fish-meal was extracted with fat solvents, no cure resulted.

It had been suspected earlier that a vitamin deficiency caused haemorrhage, and in 1934, Dam, of Copenhagen, suggested that haemorrhagic disease resulted from the lack of a fat-soluble vitamin which he named 'K' after the word 'koagulation'.

Many attempts were made to isolate the vitamin in pure form, and this was finally achieved in 1939 by Karrer, Dam and co-workers, who obtained it in a yellow oil. Two natural forms, namely, K_1 and K_2, were identified.

Sources

Vitamin K is well distributed in green plants: alfalfa (lucerne) and spinach are rich sources of supply, but vitamin K is also fairly well supplied in cauliflower, cabbage, carrot tops, kale, soya beans, seaweed and pine needles. It is present in smaller amounts in cereals, tomatoes, honey, orange peel and bran. Most of the vitamin K occurs in the green parts of the plant. Some vitamin K occurs in egg yolk, but most animal sources are only comparable with the poorest vegetable sources. However, there is very little vitamin K in potatoes, lemon juice, most fruits, or in cod liver oil.

Without vitamin K, blood will not coagulate, but the vitamin will not arrest haemorrhage, either in normal persons, or those suffering from haemophilia (a sex-linked hereditary bleeding disease occurring in males).

The sole function of vitamin K is thought to be that of a coenzyme in the liver, to help in forming prothrombin, a water-soluble protein in blood plasma. Vitamin K is stored in the liver but only in small amounts.

The coagulation of the blood is the result of a most complicated series of reactions involving prothrombin, thromboplastin, calcium, thrombin, fibrinogen, and fibrin. The actual clotting process is due to a fibrous protein called fibrin, which does not form called fibrinogen. Prothrombin in the living blood is converted to an enzyme called thrombin in shed blood. Thrombin, in the presence of calcium and the blood platelets, converts the inactive protein, fibrinogen, into fibrin. The blood clot contains corpuscles which become entangled in a web of fibrin, thus sealing off the wound and preventing further blood loss.

The precursor of thrombin, namely, prothrombin, is formed in the liver. In serious liver illness or injury, the prothrombin level in the blood falls and can endanger blood clotting.

Requirement

Human requirements of vitamin K are as yet unknown, but dietary deficiencies of this vitamin have been reported. Some vitamin K is produced by bacteria in the large intestine, but the amount is quite inadequate and must be supplemented by a dietary source of supply. The use of unsaturated fatty acids enables intestinal bacteria to synthesize vitamin K.

The new-born infant, during the first few days of its life, requires a supply of vitamin K from external sources, because the prothrombin level falls after birth and only returns to normal at the beginning of the second week, due to bacterial action.

Newly born babies are, therefore, subject to haemorrhage (which may occur from accidental minor injuries to blood vessels) while there is a lack of vitamin K. This can be due to two causes — low vitamin levels in the milk and an immature intestine in which the bacterial population, that produces vitamin K, is not sufficiently developed.

Brain haemorrhage can cause spastic paralysis in which the muscular movements are unco-ordinated and jerky, and the infant is handicapped for life. For this reason, most modern hospitals give vitamin K to the mother shortly before the baby is born. The vitamin passes from the mother's to the infant's bloodstream.

Experiments with animals have shown that a rise in temperature increases the requirements of vitamin K. A deficiency of this vitamin can be produced by the use of sulpha drugs, the salicylates, aspirin and powerful antibiotics. These together with the sulpha drugs destroy the friendly intestinal bacteria that normally produce vitamin K and so induce a deficiency.

Causes of Deficiency

An inadequate absorption of vitamin K can result from a lack of bile, pancreatic insufficiency, severe or chronic diarrhoea, ulcerative colitis, intestinal obstruction, etc.

If gallstones obstruct the bile duct, the flow of bile is shut off. Sometimes the bile duct itself becomes infected, swells and closes. In the absence of bile, natural vitamin K cannot be absorbed by the intestine. This causes a lack of prothrombin and the blood may fail to clot. Synthetic vitamin K, being water soluble, does not need bile salts for its absorption.

Vitamin K is unaffected either by the air or heat, therefore leafy vegetables can be used raw in salads or cooked, as a source of this vitamin.

9

Vitamin P (Bioflavonoids)

The term, bioflavonoids, refers to flavonoids possessing biological activity. The bioflavonoids are a group of carbon-hydrogen-oxygen compounds which have the property of correcting fragile capillaries and protecting their integrity. When bioflavonoids are lacking in the diet, the walls of blood vessels become porous and the red corpuscles can pass through them into the tissues, giving rise to several ailments.

The capillaries are so fine and so numerous that if the capillaries of one man were stretched out in a single line, they would reach two and a half times around the earth! We have mentioned elsewhere that the capillaries form an important part of the body's transport system and convey food, oxygen and hormones to every cell in the body, as well as removing the waste products of metabolism and disease. When the capillaries are strong and healthy, infections are quickly thrown off.

There is a growing recognition that because the capillaries are harmed in every diseased condition, there is no diseased state that cannot be helped tremendously by strengthening the capillaries.

The history of vitamin P began in 1926 when Gyorgyi and co-workers found that a substance extracted from paprika (red pepper) and also from lemon juice, was superior to vitamin C in preventing capillary bleeding.

Gyorgyi named this active substance 'citrin' and research revealed that it contained the bioflavonoids hesperidin, and the glycoside of eriodictyol. Later, other bioflavonoids were found, namely, quercitrin, quercetin, naringin, esculin, and hesperidin methyl chalcone. In 1944, another bioflavonoid, called rutin, was discovered by Griffith. Of those mentioned, hesperidin and rutin appear to possess the greatest biological activity. Rutin is obtained from a herb called buckwheat and also from eucalyptus. Vitamin P may, therefore, be regarded as a complex, similar to vitamin B complex.

Sources

The richest source of vitamin P is fruits, particularly lemons and oranges. It is in the inedible pulp and peel of these fruits, rather than the edible fruit, that vitamin is contained. Vitamin P is also found in rose hips, blackcurrants, grapes and buckwheat.

Gyorgyi named vitamin P 'in honour of paprika and permeability', on which latter it was found to have a profound influence.

Vitamin P is readily leached out if foods containing it are cooked in water and the water is poured away. If, however, lemon peel is added to lemonade and allowed to soak, vitamin P is extracted.

Requirement

The exact human requirement of this vitamin is not known, but is approximately 50 to 100 mg daily.

Tests have shown that vitamin P enhances the

biological effect of vitamin C by stabilizing the latter and protecting it against the destructive action of oxygen.

It has been shown, too, that when guinea pigs, in which scurvy has been produced, were given vitamin C, capillary fragility is improved, but still remains at a sub-normal level. When vitamin P is added to their diet, capillary integrity reaches normal level.

Vitamin P has a detoxicating action upon benzene and phenol and when used with vitamin C protects against the toxic effects of arsenical poisons. Unlike Vitamin C, vitamin P appears to play no part in the healing of wounds.

Uses of Vitamin P

It is accepted by science that vitamin P is an essential nutritional factor and that it produces a rise in capillary resistance, which cannot be obtained from vitamin C alone. Vitamin P has been used with some degree of success in diseases marked by decreased capillary resistance, namely, hypertension, rheumatic fever, diabetes, purpura, allergies, bacterial infections and toxicity arising from the use of drugs.

There is some evidence, too, that vitamin P has benefited those with rheumatism, rheumatoid arthritis, glaucoma and retinal haemorrhage, according to Bicknell and Prescott. These claims are confirmed by Martin in *Modern Nutrition in Health and Disease*.

Bioflavonoids and vitamin C have been used successfully for the common cold. A group of student nurses at Creighton University School of

Medicine, USA, were given tablets containing both vitamins P and C, and the results were checked against another group of nurses who received no vitamins.

The first group had 55 per cent fewer colds and their colds lasted only half the time of those of the second group.

B complex vitamins should also be taken, to ensure normal elimination of body wastes.

Concentrates of vitamin P now available, are many times stronger than those derived from fruits.

10

On Taking Vitamins

Davis says that the action of the B complex vitamins is synergistic, that is, they co-operate with each other and that better results are obtained by taking them together than by taking large doses of a single B complex vitamin.

However, these considerations apply only to conditions such as stress where there is an increased requirement of all the B vitamins. On the other hand some clinical conditions can induce a deficiency of a specific vitamin and the only way to overcome this is to take higher-than-normal intakes of that vitamin. Examples of this are vitamin B_6 deficiency induced by the contraceptive pill; increased requirements of vitamin B_6 a few days before menstruation; increased requirements of pantothenic acid in rheumatoid arthritis; the need for extra vitamin C to overcome respiratory infections and to help heal wounds.

Multi-vitamin preparations are available for those who need a daily minimum maintenance dosage. Those who require a therapeutic dosage to remedy some illness should realize that a sick person needs all the principal vitamins, but in daily dosages *larger* than a minimum maintenance dosage. Quigley states: 'Where a vitamin deficiency has existed over a long period of time, the dose that is given to correct the trouble must be several times larger than the maintenance dose.' For such people, separate vitamin capsules and tablets are available and should be taken together, in the recommended dosages.

According to Baker and Winckler, two English nutritional scientists writing in the *Medical Press*, there has been a tendency for tables of minimum vitamin requirements to be given official sanction and then to be repeatedly quoted as though they were final and absolute.

Index